KAPLAN®
medical

Anatomy
Coloring Book

by Stephanie McCann, M.A., and Eric Wise, M.S.

Simon & Schuster

NEW YORK · LONDON · SYDNEY · TORONTO

Kaplan Publishing
Published by Simon & Schuster
1230 Avenue of the Americas
New York, NY 10020

Contributing Editor: Richard Friedland, D.P.M.
Editorial Director: Jennifer Farthing
Editor: Larissa Shmailo
Production Manager: Michael Shevlin
Cover Design: Mark Weaver

August 2005
10 9 8 7 6 5 4 3 2 1

Manufactured in the United States of America
Published simultaneously in Canada

ISBN-13: 978-0-7432-6424-2
ISBN-10:   0-7432-6424-X

Table of Contents

Dedications

FROM STEPHANIE MCCANN:

…to my daughter, Natalie, for living through the creation of this book with me.

…to my teachers, Ranice Crosby, Director Emerita, and Gary Lees, Chairman and Director, Department of Art as Applied to Medicine, The Johns Hopkins University, for giving me my start in this wonderful career.

FROM ERIC WISE

…to my three brothers, Steve, Mike, and Phil for their love during good times and bad.

…to Ashley for her love and support.

About the Authors

Stephanie Paulnock McCann is a medical illustrator with a studio in Santa Barbara, California. She holds a B.A. in Fine Art from the University of California, Santa Cruz and an M.A. in Medical and Biological Illustration from the The Johns Hopkins University with a thesis in embryological illustration. Following graduate school, she was Chief of the Medical Illustration Department at Letterman Army Medical Center in San Francisco, where she received the Department of the Army Certificate of Achievement for exceptional meritorious service. Ms McCann designed and illustrated the cover of the monthly medical journal *Contemporary Orthopaedics* for many years, from the early eighties, through the late nineties.

Currently, Ms. McCann focuses on the creation of medical illustrations for use in textbooks, journals, product advertising, training manuals, and legal presentations, using both traditional and digital media. Her enjoyment of digital illustration led to 3D texture painting for computer graphics visual effects for film. Her work with Santa Barbara Studios can be seen in such films as *Star Trek: Insurrection*, and *Paulie: A Parrot's Tale*. Ms. McCann specializes in work that depicts the amazing beauty of the anatomy of the human body.

Since 1999, Ms. McCann has been an Instructor of Biological Illustration and Adobe Illustrator classes at Santa Barbara City College. She and her students exhibit annually at the Santa Barbara Museum of Natural History and the Step One Gallery in Carpinteria, California. Ms. McCann's work has also been exhibited at the Society of Illustrators in New York. Ms. McCann is a member of the Association of Medical Illustrators and the Guild of Natural Science Illustrators. Her work can be seen at www.stephaniemccann.com.

Eric Wise has been teaching biology for over 20 years at colleges and universities in California. He has taught numerous classes at California Polytechnic State University, Chabot College, College of the Sequoias, Yuba College, Santa Barbara City College, and University of California Santa Barbara. He received B.A. degrees in biology, botany, and French from Humboldt State University in Northern California and an M.S. in biology from California Polytechnic State University, San Luis Obispo. He initiated a cadaver program at Yuba College and has taught a diverse course load from marine biology to plant taxonomy.

Mr. Wise is currently an instructor at Santa Barbara City College where he has been for the last 15 years and has taught various classes including anatomy and physiology, ecology, physical anthropology, and botany. He is a member of the Human Anatomy and Physiology Society.

Mr. Wise was a director of a program abroad in Costa Rica in which students from Santa Barbara City College studied physical anthropology and tropical ecology. He is the author of several laboratory manuals in anatomy and physiology and enjoys gardening, swimming, music and teaching.

Contributing Editor **David Seiden** is professor of neuroscience and cell biology at the University of Medicine and Dentistry of New Jersey-Robert Wood Johnson Medical School; he also served as an assistant professor and associate professor of anatomy at that institution. Dr. Seiden was visiting associate professor of anatomy and cell biology at Harvard Medical School and is the author of *USMLE Step 1: Anatomy* published by Kaplan Medical. Dr. Seiden received his B.S. from The City College of New York and his Ph.D. from Temple University.

Introduction

Welcome to Kaplan Medical's *Anatomy Coloring Book*. We hope you like exploring and using the book. This unique resource is approachable, informative, and provides an enjoyable way to learn human anatomy.

People have been involved with learning anatomy from prehistoric times. Paintings in stone age caves 18 thousand years ago show evidence of anatomical structures in animals and, in some cases, humans.   In ancient Greece, Aristotle wrote extensively about the natural world and human structure was part of that writing. The Roman physician Galen is perhaps the most influential anatomist of ancient times. His works were used as the primary anatomical knowledge for about 1,500 years.

A major change in anatomy came with the Renaissance. Instead of relying on the texts of the ancient Greeks or Romans, a new sense of inquiry and investigation arose. Andreas Vesalius, an anatomist teaching in Italy, did detailed studies and drawings of the human body. Leonardo da Vinci's anatomical studies were not only great works of art, but were also a means of scientific exploration.

Today there are many anatomical resources available, from books to CDs to the Internet. New technologies for medical imaging such as CAT scans and MRI images give detailed understanding of the relationship of structures in the human body. On the Web you can find anatomy course outlines, images of the 1918 edition of *Gray's Anatomy*, cadaver photographs, and photomicrographs of microscopic anatomy. These different views and new technologies have deepened our knowledge of human anatomy.

We have designed this coloring book in appreciation of the incredible beauty of the human body, hoping to inspire you in your studies of anatomy. The connection of the eye and the hand in coloring the anatomical structures and filling in the names of these structures will be a valuable learning experience for you. Here's how to get the best results from your experience.

HOW TO USE THIS BOOK

This book is meant to be handled, colored, written on, and even cut up in the case of the muscle flash cards. There is no single way to use the coloring book, so choose the method that suits you best. It can be used to learn anatomical features by looking at the key at the bottom of the page, finding the corresponding letter on the illustration and writing in the term next to the letter before coloring the anatomical feature. This is a great learn-by-doing technique.

Another way to use the book is as a review of anatomical features or as a self-test tool. In this method you would examine the illustrations, try to fill in the appropriate blank in pencil, and then look at the key at the bottom of the page. Correct your errors and then color in the illustration as a way to cement your knowledge.

We have left the choice of colors up to you in most cases. There are a few instances where the choice of colors is designated by anatomical convention. Arteries are generally drawn in bright red, veins are deep blue, bile ducts are typically green, and nerves are usually yellow.

Coloring Techniques

The preferred medium for this book is colored pencils. Colored ballpoint pens and felt markers bleed through the page and obscure the fine detail, so colored pencils give the best result. You can use any of the many brands of colored pencils available. Begin using light pressure when you color. You can always go back and deepen the color as you work on the drawings. Look over each page before you begin coloring, so that you can color related structures in similar or related colors and can follow the anatomical conventions noted above.

This book is designed to use single, bold colors for each structure, but layering one color on top of another can be used to blend colors together if desired. Use the pencil to follow the contours or curves of the illustration. Keep bits of colored lead off the paper as dragging your hand over the paper can lead to streaks. If you are right-handed it is beneficial to color on the left side of the paper first. If you are left-handed then it is helpful to start on the right thus avoiding smearing the color with your hand.

Use the same color for the same structures. If there is a bone in three illustrations on one page, color that bone the same color in all three illustrations. That way you will easily find that bone and it will be reinforced not only by name and shape but by color as well.

Whatever reason you have for studying anatomy, this book will help you deepen your enjoyment and learning. We would love to hear about your experiences, so feel free to contact us. Thanks and happy coloring!

ANATOMICAL POSITION AND TERMS OF DIRECTION

When studying the human body it is important to place the body in anatomical position. **Anatomical position** is described as the body facing you, feet placed together and flat on the floor. The head is held erect, arms straight by the side with palms facing forward. All references to the body are made as if the body is in this position so when you describe something as being above something else it is always with respect to the body being in anatomical position.

The relative position of the parts of the human body has specific terms. **Superior** means above while **inferior** means below. **Medial** refers to being close to the midline while **lateral** means to the side. **Anterior** or **ventral** is to the front while **posterior** or **dorsal** is to the back. Superficial is near the surface while deep means to the core of the body. When working with the limbs, **proximal** means closer to the trunk while **distal** is to the ends of the extremities. Write the directional terms in the spaces provided and color in the arrows in reference to these terms. Note that these terms are somewhat different for four legged animals.

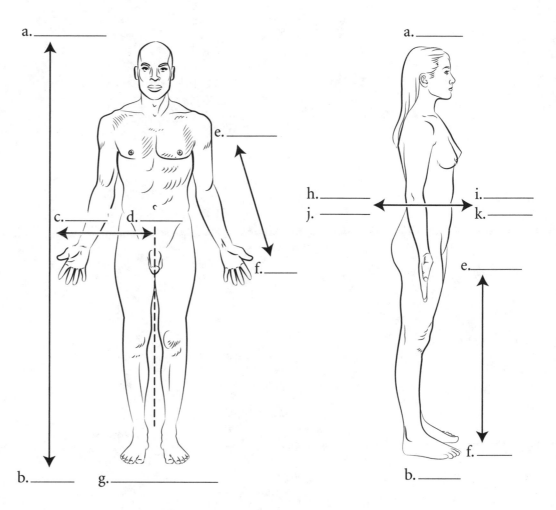

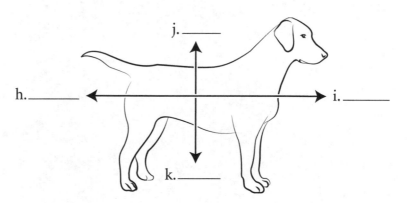

Answer Key: a. Superior, b. Inferior, c. Lateral, d. Medial, e. Proximal, f. Distal, g. Anatomical position, h. Posterior, i. Anterior, j. Dorsal, k. Ventral

ANATOMICAL PLANES OF THE BODY

Many specimens in anatomy are sectioned so that the interior of the organ or region can be examined. It is important that the direction of the cut is known so that the proper orientation of the specimen is known. A heart looks very different if it is cut along its length as opposed to horizontally. A horizontal cut is known as a **transverse section** or a **cross section**. A cut that divides the body or an organ into anterior and posterior parts is a **coronal section** or **frontal section**. One that divides the structure into left and right parts is a **sagittal section**. If the body is divided directly down the middle the section is known as a **midsagittal section**. A midsagittal section is usually reserved for dividing the body into to equal left and right parts. If an organ (such as the eye) is sectioned into two equal parts such that there is a left and right half then this is known as a **median section**. Label the illustrations and color in the appropriate planes.

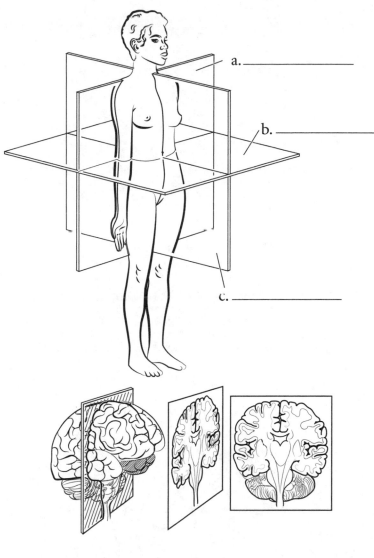

a. _____

b. _____

c. _____

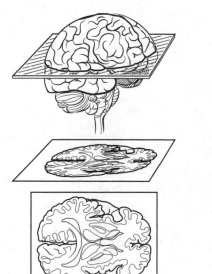
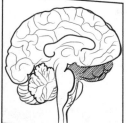

a. _____

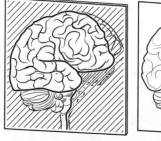
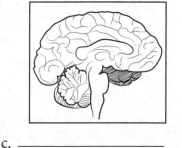

b. _____   c. _____

HIERARCHY OF THE BODY

The human body can be studied at different levels. Organs such as the stomach can be grouped into organ systems (digestive system) or can be studied on a smaller scale like the cellular level. The ranking of these levels is called a **hierarchy**. The smallest organizational unit is the **atom**. Individual atoms are grouped into larger structures called **molecules**.

These in turn make up **organelles**, which are part of a larger, more complicated systems called **cells**. Cells are the structural and functional units of life. Cells are clustered into **tissues**. **Organs** are discreet units made up of two or more tissues and organs are grouped into **organ systems** that compose the **organism**. Label the levels of the hierarchy and color each item a different color.

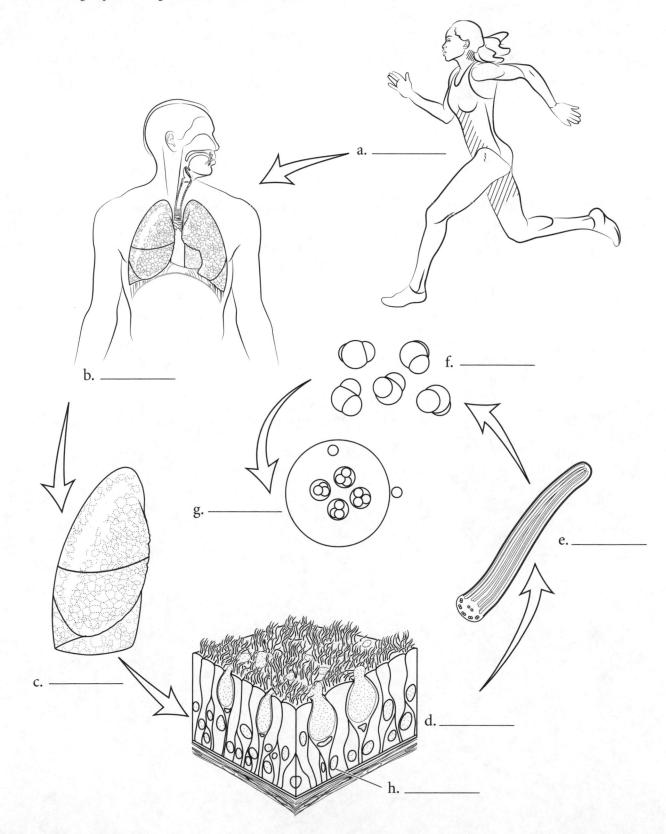

a. _____

b. _____

c. _____

d. _____

e. _____

f. _____

g. _____

h. _____

Answer Key: a. Organism (human), b. Organ system (respiratory system) c. Organ (lung), d. Tissue (epithelium), e. Organelle (cilia), f. Molecule, g. Atom, h. cells

REGIONS OF THE ABDOMEN

In anatomy the abdomen is divided into nine regions. Write the names of the regions in the spaces indicated. Color both the left and right **hypochondriac** regions in light blue. Hypochondriac means "below the cartilage." The common use of the word (someone who thinks they are sick all the time) reflects the Greek origin of the word as the ancient Greeks considered the region to be the center of sadness. Inferior to the hypochondriac regions are the **lumbar** or **lateral abdominal** regions. These are commonly known as the "love handles." Use yellow for these regions. Below the lumbar regions are the **inguinal** or **iliac** regions. You should color in these regions with the same shade of green. In the middle of the abdomen is the **umbilical** region. Color this region in red. Above this is the **epigastric** region (*epi* = above and *gastric* = stomach). Color this region in purple. Below the umbilical region is the **hypogastric** region (*hypo* = below). Color this region in a darker blue.

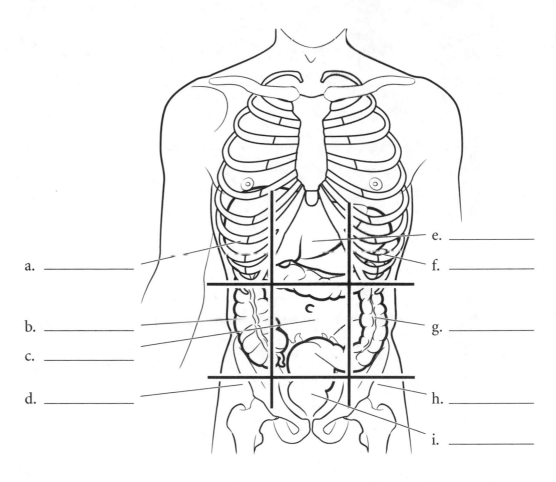

a. _____

b. _____

c. _____

d. _____

e. _____

f. _____

g. _____

h. _____

i. _____

In clinical settings a quadrant approach is used. Write the names of the regions (**right upper quadrant, left upper quadrant, right lower quadrant, left lower quadrant**) in the spaces provided. Color each quadrant a different color.

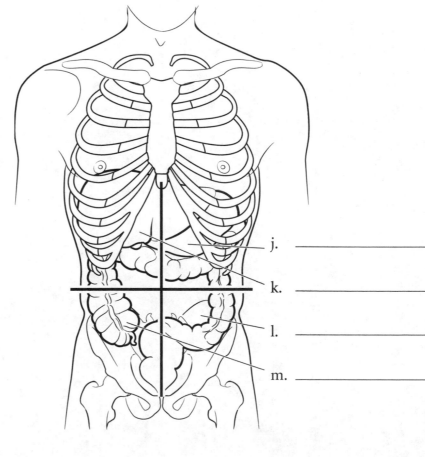

j. _____

k. _____

l. _____

m. _____

Answer Key: a Right hypochondriac, b. Right lumbar (lateral abdominal), c. Umbilical, d. Right inguinal or iliac, e. Epigastric, f. Left hypochondriac, g. Left lumbar (lateral abdominal), h. Left inguinal or iliac, i. Hypogastric, j. Left upper quadrant, k. Right upper quadrant, l. Left lower quadrant, m. Right lower quadrant

ORGAN SYSTEMS

The human body is either studied by regions or by organs systems. This book uses the organ system approach in which individual organs (such as bones) are grouped into the larger organ system (for example, the skeletal system). Typically eleven organ systems are described. The **skeletal system** consists of all of the bones of the body. Examples are the **femur** and the **humerus**. The **nervous system** consists of the **nerves, spinal cord,** and **brain** while the **lymphatic system** consists of **lymph glands**, conducting tubes called **lymphatics**, and organs such as the **spleen**. The term immune system is more of a functional classification and will not be treated as a separate system here. The **muscular system** consists of individual skeletal muscles as organs such as the **pectoralis major** and **deltoid**. Label the organ systems underneath each illustration and label the selected organs by using the terms available. When you finish, select different colors for each organ system and color them in.

Organ System	Organ	Organ	Organ
Skeletal system	Femur	Humerus	
Nervous system	Nerves	Spinal cord	Brain
Lymphatic system	Lymph glands	Spleen	
Muscular system	Pectoralis major	Deltoid	

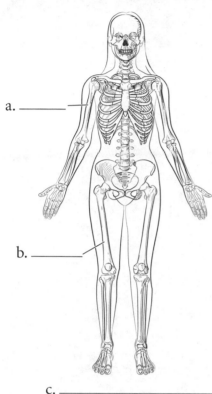

a. _____
b. _____
c. _____

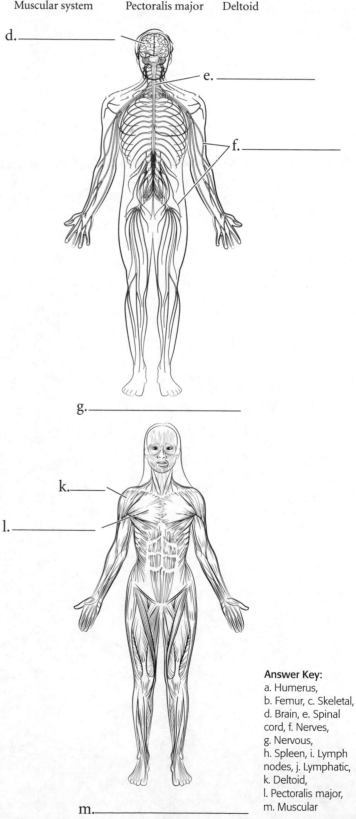

d. _____
e. _____
f. _____
g. _____

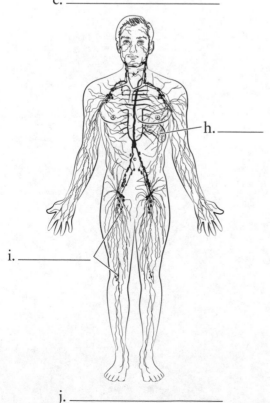

h. _____
i. _____
j. _____

k. _____
l. _____
m. _____

Answer Key:
a. Humerus, b. Femur, c. Skeletal, d. Brain, e. Spinal cord, f. Nerves, g. Nervous, h. Spleen, i. Lymph nodes, j. Lymphatic, k. Deltoid, l. Pectoralis major, m. Muscular

ORGAN SYSTEMS (CONTINUED)

The **skin** and other structures are in the **integumentary system** and the **digestive system** involves the breakdown and absorption of food with organs such as the **esophagus** and **stomach**. The **endocrine system** is made of the glands that secrete hormones such as the **thyroid gland** and the **adrenal glands**. The **respiratory system** involves the transfer of oxygen and carbon dioxide between the air and the blood. The respiratory system consists of organs such as the **trachea** and **lungs**.

Label the organ systems underneath each illustration and label the selected organs by using the terms available. When you finish, select different colors for each organ system and color them in.

Organ System	**Organ**	**Organ**
Integumentary system	Skin	
Digestive system	Esophagus	Stomach
Endocrine system	Thyroid gland	Adrenal glands
Respiratory system	Trachea	Lungs

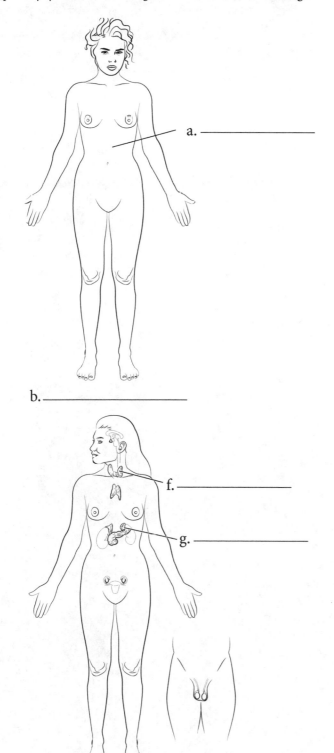

a. _____

b. _____

h. _____

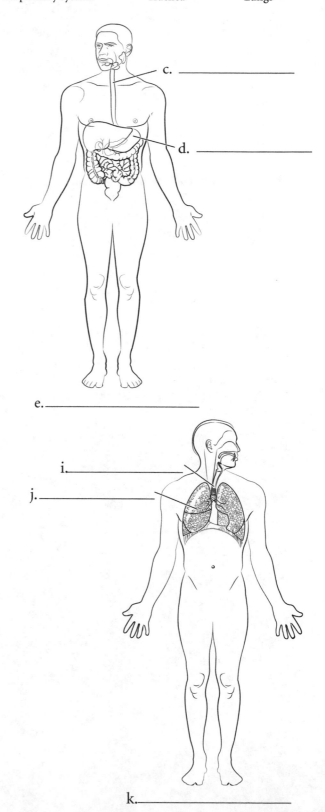

c. _____

d. _____

e. _____

i. _____

j. _____

k. _____

Answer Key: a. Skin, b. Integumentary, c. Esophagus, d. Stomach, e. Digestive, f. Thyroid gland, g. Adrenal gland, h. Endocrine, i. Trachea, j. Lung, k. Respiratory

ORGAN SYSTEMS (CONTINUED)

The **heart** and associated **blood vessels** compose the **cardiovascular system** which circulates blood throughout the body. The **urinary system** filters, stores, and conducts some wastes from the body. The **bladder** and **urethra** are part of the **urinary system.** The **testes** and **ovaries** are part of the **reproductive system** and this system perpetuates the species. The differentiation of male and female systems makes this organ system unique among the other systems. These eleven organs systems can be remembered by the memory clue **LN Cries Drum**. Each letter represents

the first letter of a name of an organ system. Label the organ systems underneath each illustration and label the selected organs by using the terms available. When you finish, select different colors for each organ system and color them in.

Organ System	**Organ**	**Organ**
Cardiovascular system	Heart	Blood vessels
Urinary system	Bladder	Urethra
Reproductive system	Testes	Ovaries

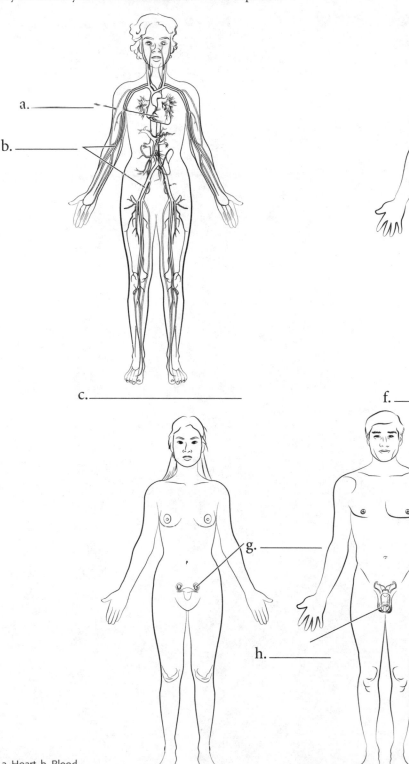

a. _____
b. _____
c. _____
d. _____
e. _____
f. _____
g. _____
h. _____
i. _____

Answer Key: a. Heart, b. Blood vessels, c. Cardiovascular, d. Bladder, e. Urethra, f. Urinary, g. Ovary, h. Testis, i. Reproductive

BODY REGIONS (ANTERIOR)

There are specific anatomical terms for regions of the body. These areas or regions frequently have Greek or Latin names because early western studies in anatomy occurred in Greece and Rome. During the Renaissance, European scholars studied anatomy and applied the ancient names to the structures. Label the various regions of the body and fill in their names. You can use a standard anatomy text or follow the key at the bottom of the page. A list of terms and their common names follows for the anterior side of the body. Color in the regions of the body.

cranial (head)
facial (face)
cervical (neck)
deltoid (shoulder)
pectoral (chest)
sternal (center of chest)
brachial (arm)
antebrachial (forearm)
manual (hand)
digital (fingers)
abdominal (belly)
inguinal (groin)
coxal (hip)
femoral (thigh)
genicular (knee)
crural (leg)
pedal (foot)
digital (toes)

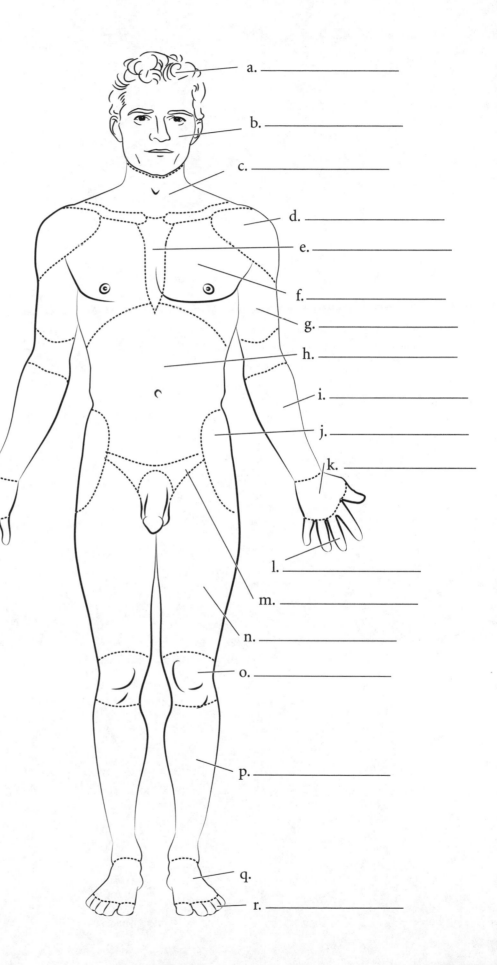

a. _____
b. _____
c. _____
d. _____
e. _____
f. _____
g. _____
h. _____
i. _____
j. _____
k. _____
l. _____
m. _____
n. _____
o. _____
p. _____
q. _____
r. _____

Answer Key: a. Cranial (head), b. Facial (face), c. Cervical (neck), d. Deltoid (shoulder), e. Sternal (center of chest), f. Pectoral (chest), g. Brachial (arm), h. Abdominal (belly), i. Antebrachial (forearm), j. Coxal (hip), k. Manual (hand), l. Digital (fingers), m. Inguinal, n. Femoral (thigh), o. Genicular (knee), p. Crural (leg), q. Pedal (foot), r. Digital (toes)

BODY REGIONS (POSTERIOR)

For the posterior view of the body fill in the terms and color the regions of the body. The anatomical names are given first with the common names in parentheses.

cephalic (head)
nuchal (neck)
scapular (shoulder blade)
vertebral (backbone)
lumbar (love handles)
brachial (arm)
olecranon (elbow)
antebrachial (forearm)
gluteal (buttocks)
femoral (thigh)
popliteal (back of knee)
sural (calf)
calcaneal (heel)

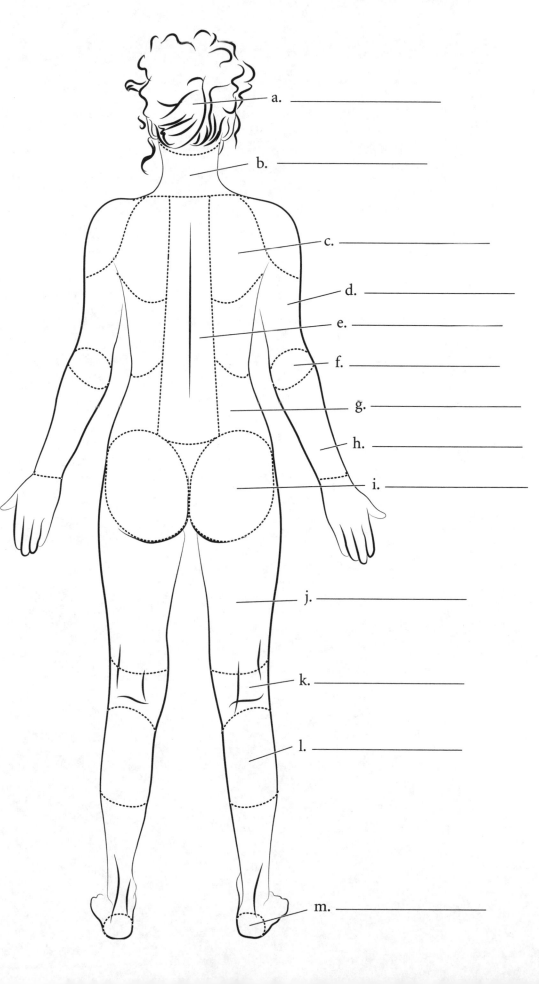

a. _____

b. _____

c. _____

d. _____

e. _____

f. _____

g. _____

h. _____

i. _____

j. _____

k. _____

l. _____

m. _____

Answer Key: a.Cephalic (head), b. Nuchal (neck), c. Scapular (shoulder blade), d. Brachial (arm), e. Vertebral (backbone), f. Olecranon (elbow), g. Lumbar (love handles), h. Antebrachial (forearm), i. Gluteal (buttocks), j. Femoral (thigh), k. Popliteal (back of knee), l. Sural (calf), m. Calcaneal (heel)

BODY CAVITIES

The organs of the body are frequently found in body cavities. The body is divided into two main cavities, the **dorsal body cavity** and the **ventral body cavity**. The dorsal body cavity consists of the **cranial cavity,** which houses the brain and the **spinal canal,** which surrounds the spinal cord. The ventral body cavity contains the upper **thoracic cavity,** which is subdivided into the **pleural cavities,** housing the lungs, and the **mediastinum.** The mediastinum contains the heart in the **pericardial cavity,** the major vessels near the heart, nerves, and the esophagus. Below the thoracic cavity is the **abdominopelvic cavity,** which contains the upper **abdominal cavity,** housing the digestive organs, and the inferior **pelvic cavity,** which holds the uterus and rectum in females or just the rectum in males. Label the specific and major cavities of the body and color them with different colors.

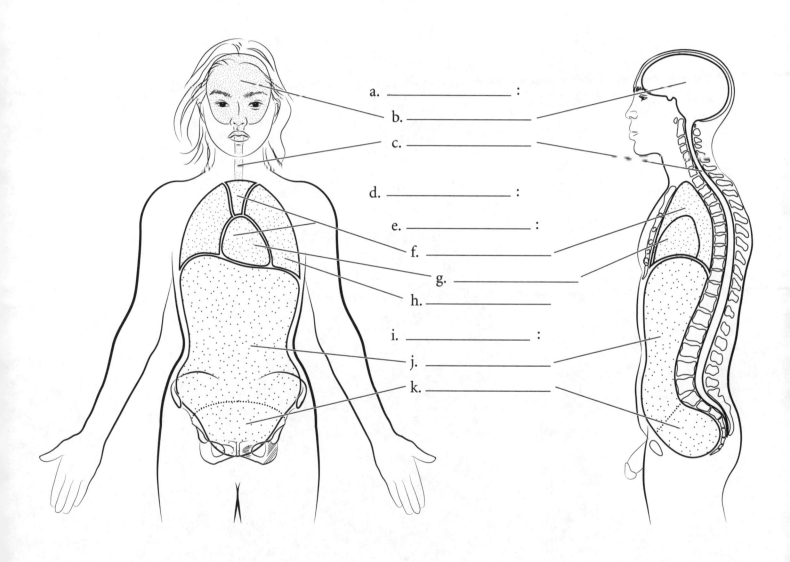

a. _____ :

b. _____

c. _____

d. _____ :

e. _____ :

f. _____

g. _____

h. _____

i. _____ :

j. _____

k. _____

Answer Key: a. Dorsal body cavity, b. Cranial cavity, c. Spinal canal, d. Ventral body cavity, e. Thoracic cavity, f. Mediastinum, g. Pericardial cavity, h. Pleural cavity, i. Abdominopelvic cavity, j. Abdominal cavity, k. Pelvic cavity

OVERVIEW OF CELL AND CELL MEMBRANE

Cells consist of an enclosing **plasma membrane**, an inner **cytoplasm** with numerous **organelles**, and other cellular structures. The fluid portion of the cell is called the **cytosol**. Color the cytosol in last after you color the rest of the cellular structures. One of the major structures in the cell is the **nucleus**. It is the genetic center of the cell and consists of fluid **karyoplasm**, **chromatin** (containing DNA), and the **nucleolus**. Color these features and label them on the illustration.

The **cytoskeleton** consists of microtubules, intermediate filaments and microfilaments. It is involved in maintaining cell shape, fixing organelles, and directing some cellular activity.

Label the organelles of the cell and use a different color for each one. The **mitochondria** are the energy-producing structures of the cell while the

Golgi apparatus assembles complex biomolecules and transports them out of the cell. Proteins are made in the cell by ribosomes. If the ribosomes are found by themselves in the cytoplasm, they are called **free ribosomes**. If they are attached to the **rough endoplasmic reticulum**, they are called **bound ribosomes**. The **smooth endoplasmic reticulum** manufactures lipids and helps in breaking down toxic materials in the cell. Other structures in the cell are **vesicles** (sacs that hold liquids). **Phagocytic vesicles** ingest material into the cell. **Lysosomes** contain digestive enzymes while **peroxisomes** degrade hydrogen peroxide in the cell. After you label and color the organelles make sure to go back and shade in the cytosol. **Centrioles** are microtubules grouped together and are involved in cell division.

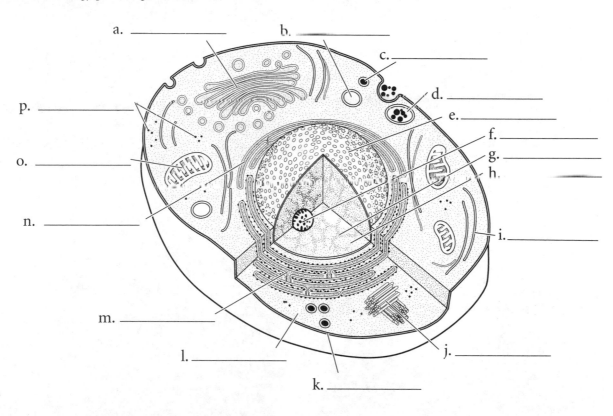

The **plasma membrane** is composed of a **phospholipid bilayer**. Color the **phosphate molecules** on the outside and inside of the membrane one color and the **lipid layer** another color. **Cholesterol molecules** occur in the membrane and, depending on their concentration, can make the membrane stiff or more fluid. Proteins that are found on the outside of the membrane are called **peripheral proteins** while proteins that pass

through the membrane are called **integral proteins**. Frequently these make up gates or channels that allow material to pass through the membrane. Attached to proteins on the cell membrane are **carbohydrate chains**. These provide cellular identity. Label and color the cell membrane structures.

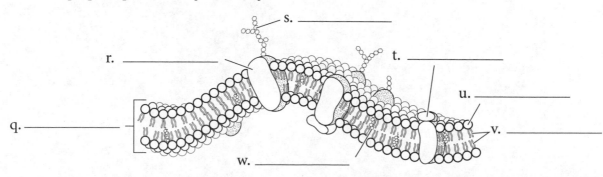

Answer Key: a. Golgi apparatus, b. Lysosome, c. Peroxisome, d. Phagocytic vesicle, e. Nucleus, f. Nucleolus, g. Chromatin, h. Karyoplasm, i. Cytoskeleton, j. Centrioles, k. Plasma membrane, l. Cytoplasm, m. Rough endoplasmic reticulum, n. Smooth endoplasmic reticulum, o. Mitochondrion, p. Free ribosomes, q. Phospholipid bilayer, r. Integral protein, s. Carbohydrate chain, t. Peripheral protein, u. Phosphate molecule, v. Lipid layer, w. Cholesterol molecule

SIMPLE EPITHELIA

There are four types of tissues in humans and these make up all of the organs and binding material in the body. **Epithelial tissue** makes up linings of the body. In many cases, where there is exposure (outside, such as the skin, or inside, such as in blood vessels), epithelium is the tissue found. It is named according to its layers (typically simple or stratified) and the shape of cells (such as cuboidal). **Simple squamous epithelium** is a single layer of flattened cells. **Simple cuboidal epithelium** is also a single layer of cells but the cells are in the shape of cubes. **Simple columnar epithelium** is a single layer of long columnar cells. Label and color these epithelial types and pay attention to the **basement membrane**, the noncellular layer that attaches the epithelium to lower layers. It should be colored red. Color the **nuclei** in purple, the **cytoplasm** blue, and label the cells.

Pseudostratified ciliated columnar epithelium is in a single layer of cells but it looks stratified on first appearance. Not all of the cells reach the surface of the tissue. All of the cells reach the basement membrane. Label and color the **nuclei**, **basement membrane**, **cell membrane** and the **cilia** in this tissue.

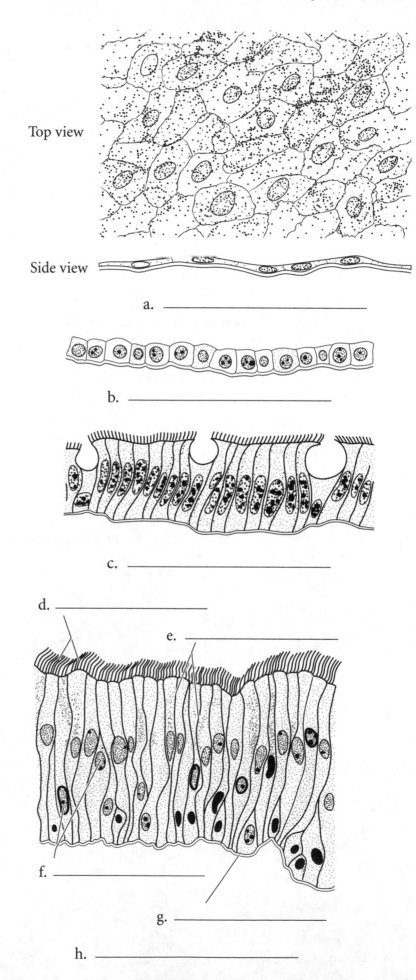

Top view

Side view

a. _____

b. _____

c. _____

d. _____

e. _____

f. _____

g. _____

h. _____

Answer Key: a. Simple squamous epithelium, b. Simple cuboidal epithelium, c. Simple columnar epithelium, d. Cilia, e. Cell membrane, f. Nuclei, g. Basement membrane, h. Pseudostratified ciliated columnar epithelium

STRATIFIED EPITHELIA

There are two common epithelial tissues that are many-layered. **Stratified squamous epithelium** is many layers of flattened cells. Label and color the basement membrane red, color the cytoplasm blue, and the nuclei purple. There are two major types of stratified squamous epithelium. Keratinized epithelium is found on the skin and is toughened by the protein keratin. Non-keratinized stratified squamous epithelium is found in the oral cavity and vagina and is a mucous membrane.

Another main type of layered epithelial tissue is **transitional epithelium**. This is tissue that lines part of the urinary tract including the bladder. When the bladder is empty, the cells bunch up on one another and the tissue is thick. When the bladder is full, the cells stretch out into a few layers. Label the cell types for each picture and color the structures in the same way as in previous illustrations.

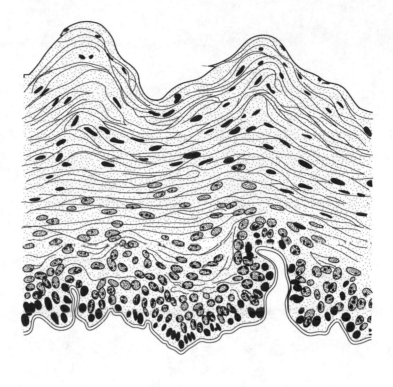

a. _____

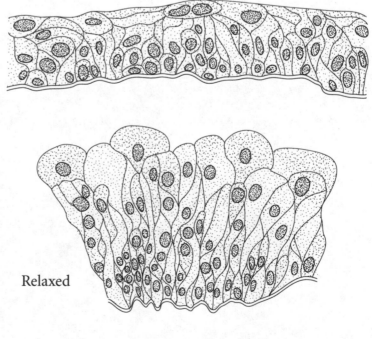

Stretched

Relaxed

b. _____

GLANDS

There are several types of glands in the human body. Some of these glands secrete their products into tubes or ducts. These are known as **exocrine** glands. Other glands secrete their products into the spaces between cells where they are picked up by the blood or lymph system. These are the **endocrine** glands. Endocrine glands secrete hormones that have an impact on target tissues of the body.

Glands can be unicellular or multicellular. Glands that consist of just one cell are called **goblet cells**. They secrete mucus, which is a lubricant. There are many types of multicellular glands. They are classified by how they secrete their products. Some glands secrete products from **vesicles** pinched off from the cell. These are called **merocine** glands. In these glands no cellular material is lost in the secretion of material. An example of a merocrine gland is a sweat gland. Some cells squeeze parts of the cell off to secrete cellular products. These are known as **apocrine** glands. The lactiferous glands that produce milk are apocrine glands. Some secretions occur by the entire cell rupturing. These are called **holocrine** glands. Oil glands of the skin are holocrine glands. Label the glands and color them in on the figure.

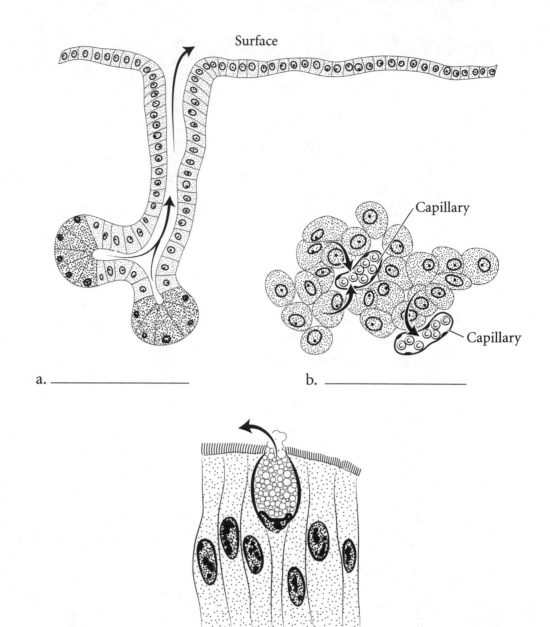

Surface

a. _____

b. _____

Capillary

Capillary

c. _____

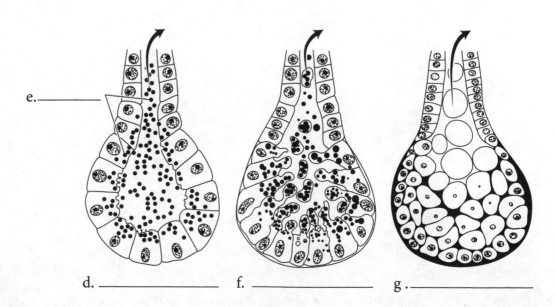

e.

d. _____   f. _____   g. _____

Answer Key: a. Exocrine gland,
b. Endocrine gland, c. Goblet cell,
d. Merocrine glands, e. Vesicles,
f. Apocrine glands, g. Holocrine glands

CONNECTIVE TISSUE

Connective tissue is a varied group of associated tissues, all of which are derived from an embryonic tissue known as mesenchyme. Connective tissue not only has cells, as do all of the other tissues, but it also has **fibers** and a large amount of background substance called **matrix**. There are many specific tissues that belong to connective tissue. **Loose connective tissue** is found wrapping around organs or under the epidermis and it is composed of **collagenous**, **elastic**, and **reticular fibers**, a liquid matrix and numerous cells, many of which have an immune function. **Dense regular connective tissue** has a few cells called **fibrocytes** and a small amount of matrix with most of the tissue composed of a regular arrangement of **collagenous fibers**. This specific tissue makes up tendons and ligaments. If the fibers are not in an orderly arrangement, then the tissue is called **dense irregular connective tissue**. This tissue is found in places like the white of the eye.

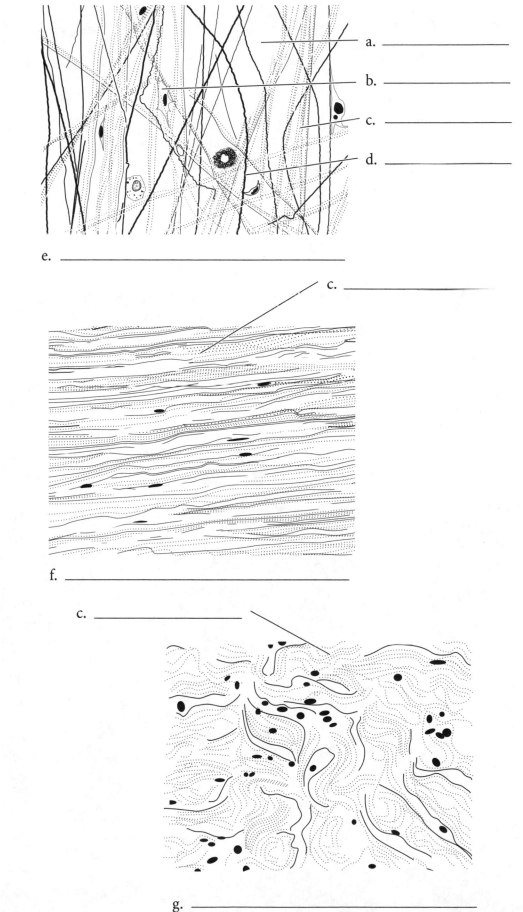

a. _____

b. _____

c. _____

d. _____

e. _____

c. _____

f. _____

c. _____

g. _____

CONNECTIVE TISSUE (CONTINUED)

Elastic connective tissue contains **elastic fibers** and is found in areas that recoil when stretched such as in the walls of arteries. **Reticular connective tissue** consists of **reticular fibers** that form an internal support in soft organs such as the liver and spleen. **Adipose tissue** consists of specialized fat-storing cells called adipocytes. Label and color the components of these connective tissues.

a. _____   b. _____

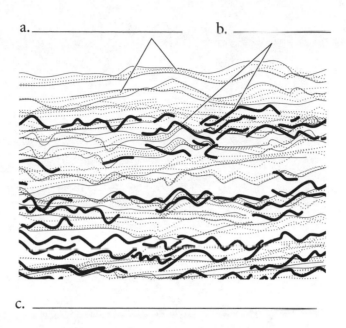

c. _____

d. _____

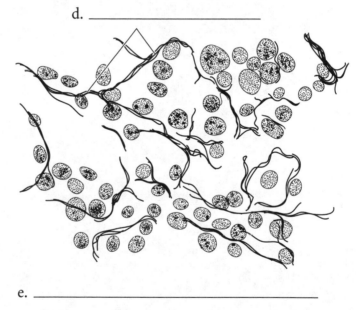

e. _____

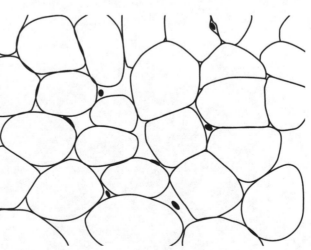

f. _____

Answer Key: a. Collagenous fibers, b. Elastic fibers, c. Elastic connective tissue, d. Reticular fibers, e. Reticular connective tissue, f. Adipose tissue

CARTILAGE

There are three types of cartilage in connective tissue. The most common kind of cartilage is **hyaline cartilage**. It contains a semisolid **matrix**, **collagenous fibers**, and **chondrocytes** (cartilage cells). The end of the nose is pliable due to hyaline cartilage. **Fibrocartilage** is like hyaline cartilage, having the same components, but there are more collagenous fibers in fibrocartilage. It is found in areas where there is more stress, such as the joint between the bones of the thigh and leg. **Elastic cartilage** has a matrix, chondrocytes, and **elastic fibers**. These fibers make the cartilage more bendable than hyaline cartilage. Label and color the cells and fibers of cartilage and use a light color to shade the matrix such as a pale pink or blue.

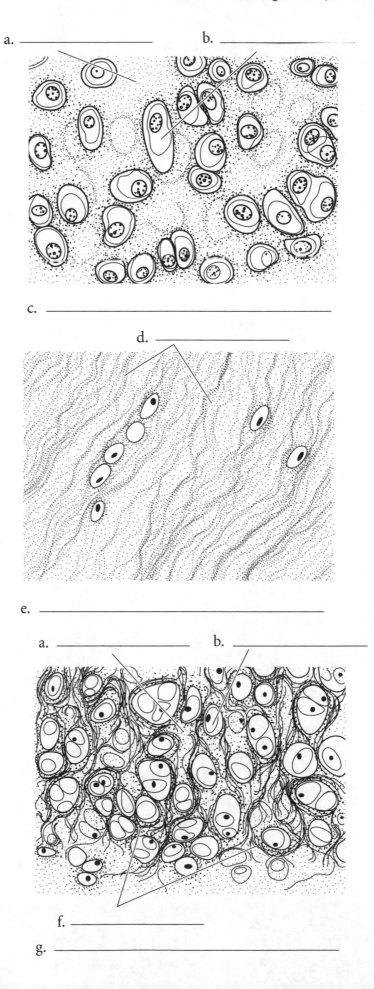

a. _____ b. _____

c. _____

d. _____

e. _____

a. _____ b. _____

f. _____

g. _____

Answer Key: a. Matrix, b. Chondrocytes, c. Hyaline cartilage, d. Collagenous fibers, e. Fibrocartilage, f. Elastic fibers, g. Elastic cartilage

BONE AND BLOOD

Bone is a connective tissue. The cells are the **osteocytes** and the fibers are collagenous fibers enclosed in a hard matrix of bone salts. You will not see the fibers in the illustration because they are covered by the dense matrix. Label and color the osteocytes and matrix of bone.

Blood is another kind of connective tissue. The matrix in blood is the **plasma** and the cells are **erythrocytes** (red blood cells) and **leukocytes** (white blood cells).

Platelets are small flat disks in the blood that aid in clotting.

a. _____

b. _____

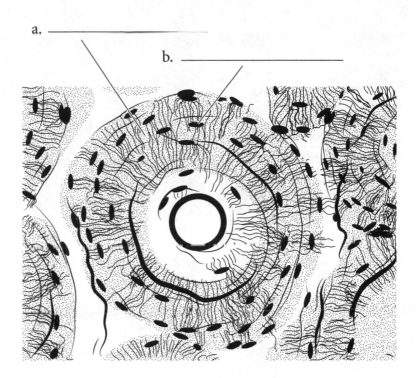

c. _____

d. _____   e. _____

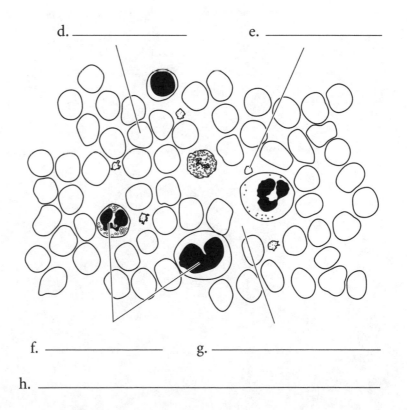

f. _____   g. _____

h. _____

Answer Key: a. Matrix, b. Osteocyte.
c. Bone, d. Erythrocyte, e. Platelet,
f. Leukocytes, g. Plasma, h. Blood

MUSCLE AND NERVOUS TISSUE

Muscular tissue is composed of specialized cells involved in contraction. **Skeletal muscle** makes up body muscles and represents around 40 percent of the body mass. Skeletal muscle is striated and the fusion of individual cells produces longer, mature cells that are multinucleate. These nuclei are found on the edges of the cells. Skeletal muscle can be consciously controlled and is called voluntary muscle. Label and color the **striations** of the skeletal muscle cells, the **nuclei**, and individual **cells**.

Cardiac muscle is also **striated** but the striations are not as obvious as in skeletal muscle. This muscle is found in the heart and is involuntary. It does not involve conscious control. Cardiac muscle typically has only one centrally located **nucleus** per cell, and the cells themselves are branched. They attach to other cells by **intercalated discs**, which allow communication between cells for the conduction of impulses during the cardiac cycle. Label and color these features on the illustration.

Smooth muscle is not striated and it is involuntary. The cells are slender and have one nucleus located in the center of the cell. It is widely distributed in the body, making up, among other things, part of the digestive system, reproductive system, and integumentary system. Smooth muscle is found in glands and other areas not under conscious control. Label and color the **nucleus** and **cell** of smooth muscle.

Nervous tissue consists of the **neuron** and associated **glial cells**. Neurons have numerous branched extensions called **dendrites**, a central **nerve cell body** (**soma**) that houses the **nucleus**, and a long extension called an **axon**. The glial cells, also known as **neuroglia**, have many functions. Some of these are supportive of the neuron and some may involve processing of neural information. Label and color the parts of the neuron and the glial cells.

a. _____   b. _____

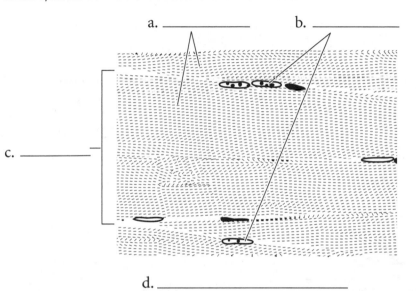

c. _____

d. _____

b. _____   e. _____

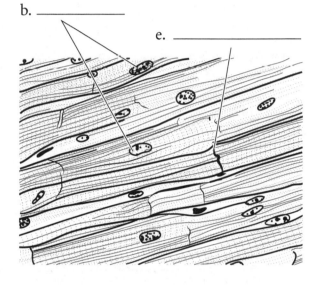

f. _____

b. _____   c. _____

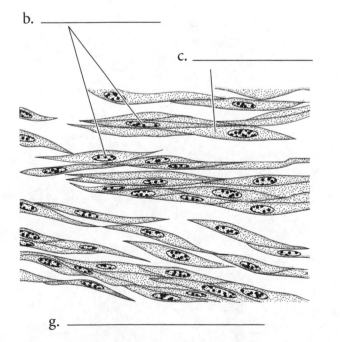

g. _____

i. _____   j. _____

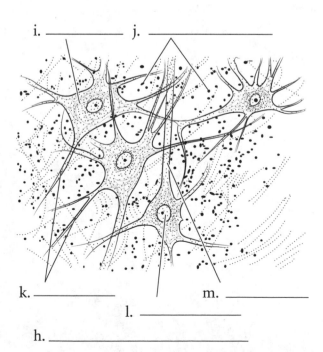

k. _____   m. _____

l. _____

h. _____

Answer Key: a. Striations, b. Nuclei, c. Cell, d. Skeletal muscle, e. Intercalated disc, f. Cardiac muscle, g. Smooth muscle, h. Nervous tissue, i. Nerve cell body, j. Glial cells (Neuroglia), k. Dendrites, l. Nucleus, m. Axon

INTEGUMENTARY SYSTEM

The most superficial layer of the skin is the epidermis. Color the five layers of the epidermis. The deepest layer is the **stratum basale** and there are specific cells called **melanocytes** that secrete the brown pigment **melanin**. Color the majority of the stratum basale pink but color the melanocytes brown. Color the **stratum spinosum** a light blue. The **stratum granulosum** has purple granules in it so color that layer using purple dots. The **stratum lucidum** (found only in thick skin) is a thin, light colored layer so yellow or white are good colors for this tissue. Color the superficial **stratum corneum** orange.

The overview of the skin contains many layers. Color the **epidermis** a red-orange. The **dermis** consists of two layers, an upper **papillary layer,** which should be colored in a light pink, and a deeper **reticular layer,** which should be colored a darker pink. There are **sweat glands** that are found in the dermis that can be colored purple. You should color the **hypodermis** (not a part of the integument) yellow because of the amount of fat found there. Two types of touch receptors can easily be seen in microscopic sections. These are the **Meissner corpuscles** and the **Pacinian corpuscles.**

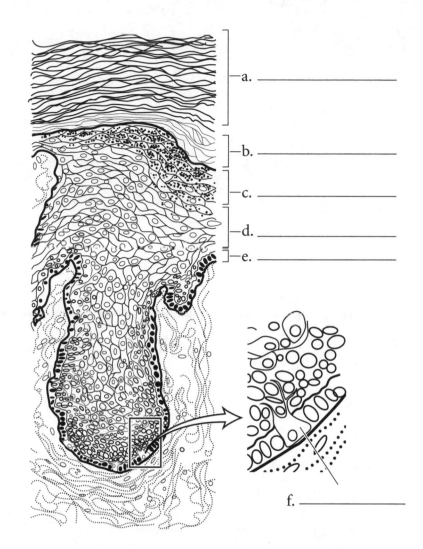

a. _____

b. _____

c. _____

d. _____

e. _____

f. _____

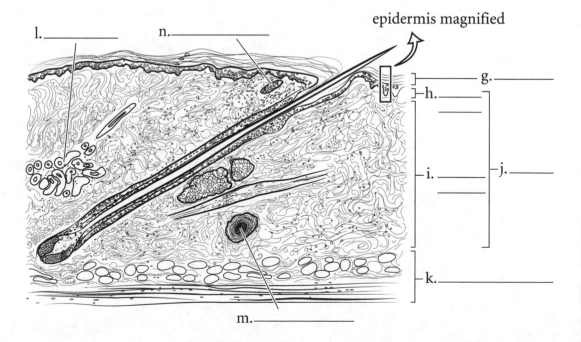

epidermis magnified

l. _____

n. _____

g. _____

h. _____

i. _____

j. _____

k. _____

m. _____

Answer Key: a. Stratum corneum, b. Stratum lucidum, c. Stratum granulosum, d. Stratum spinosum, e. Stratum basale, f. Melanocyte, g. Epidermis, h. Papillary layer, i. Reticular layer, j. Dermis, k. Hypodermis, l. Sweat gland, m. Pacinian corpuscle, n. Meissner corpuscle

HAIR AND NAILS

Hair consists of several parts. The hair originates from the dermal papilla and the deepest part of the hair is known as the **hair bulb**. The hair is pushed superficially and forms the **hair root** (the part of the hair enclosed in the skin). Once the hair erupts from the skin it is known as the **hair shaft**. Color the three sections of hair different shades of blue. The hair is enclosed by the **hair follicle**, which should be colored purple.

Associated with the hair are the **arrector pili** muscle, which is made of smooth muscle and is colored pink, and an oil-secreting gland known as the **sebaceous gland**, which should be colored yellow.

Fingernails and toenails are considered accessory structures of the integument. Color the diagram labeling the **nail plate**, the **free edge**, the **nail fold**, the **lunula**, **eponychium** (cuticle), **nail root**, **hyponychium** and the **nail bed**.

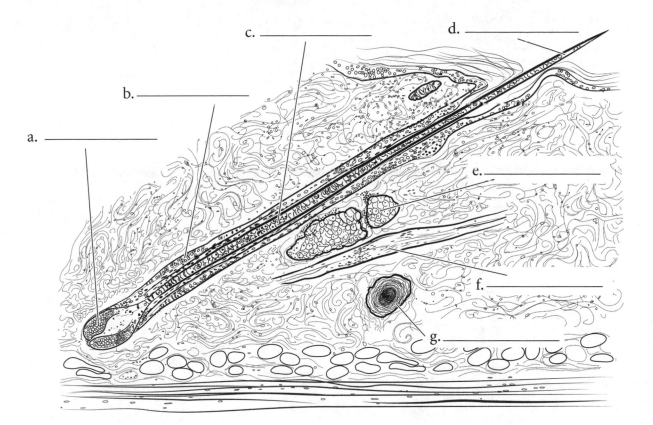

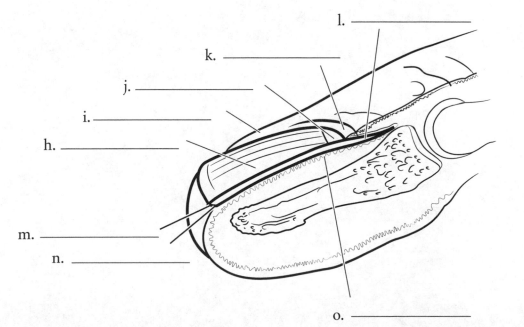

Answer Key: a. Bulb, b. Follicle, c. Root, d. Shaft, e. Sebaceous gland, f. Arrector pili. g. Pacinian corpuscle, h. Nail plate, i. Nail fold, j. Lunula, k. Eponychium, l. Nail root, m. Free edge, n. Hyponychium, o. Nail matrix (Nail bed)

FRONTAL ASPECT OF THE SKULL

The skull is a complex structure. There are 8 cranial bones and 14 facial bones in the skull. From the anterior view most of the facial bones can be seen and some of the cranial bones are visible too. The bone that makes up the forehead and extends beyond the eyebrows is the **frontal bone**. This bone forms the upper rim of the **orbit,** which is a socket that encloses the eye. In the back of the orbit is the **sphenoid bone** and the lateral walls of the orbit are composed of the **zygomatic bones.** The bridge of the nose consists of the paired **nasal bones** and just lateral to

them are the two **maxillae**. These bones hold the upper teeth. The lower teeth are held by the **mandible**. Inside the nasal cavity two projections can be seen. These are the inferior nasal conchae. The wall that divides the nasal cavity is the **nasal septum** and it consists of two bones, the ethmoid bone and the vomer. Along the side of the skull are the **temporal bones**, located posterior to the zygomatic bones. Label the major bones of the skull and color them in. As you color in the skull try to use the same color for the same bone on different pages. This will help you associate the same bone with various views from which it can be seen.

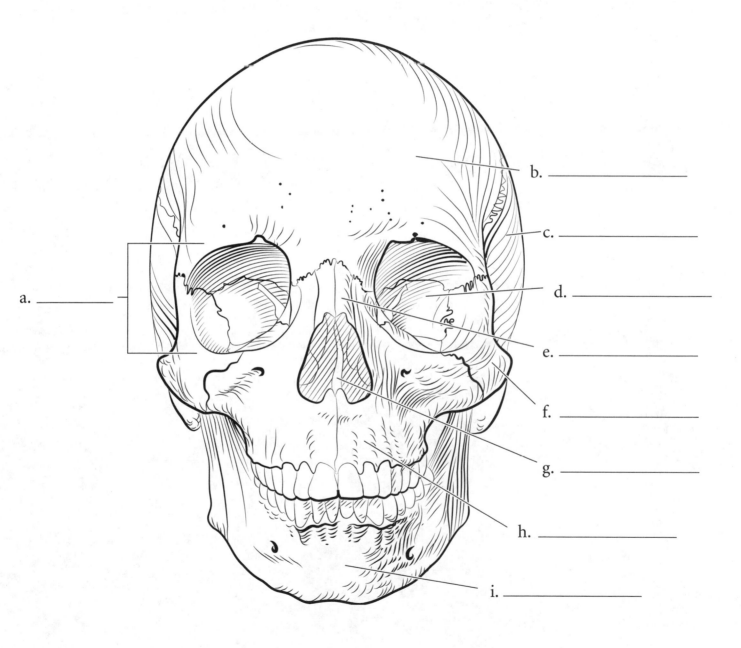

a. _____

b. _____

c. _____

d. _____

e. _____

f. _____

g. _____

h. _____

i. _____

Answer Key: a. Orbit, b. Frontal bone, c. Temporal bone, d. Sphenoid bone, e. Nasal bone, f. Zygomatic bone, g. Nasal septum, h. Maxilla, i. Mandible

LATERAL VIEW OF THE SKULL

Many bones seen from the anterior view can also be seen from the lateral view. The **frontal bone** is joined to the **parietal bones** by the **coronal suture**. The parietal bones span much of the cranium and articulate with the **occipital bone** at the **lambdoid suture**. There is a posterior extension of the **occipital bone** known as the **external occipital protuberance**. The exterior aspect of the **temporal bone** is seen from the lateral view and many of the significant features such as the **mastoid process**, **external acoustic meatus**, and **styloid process** are visible. On the side is the elongated **zygomatic process**. The temporal bone articulates with other cranial bones by the **squamous suture**. The bone anterior to the temporal bone is the **sphenoid bone**. It is a bone that is found in the middle of the skull. The **nasal bone** is visible from the lateral view and its relationship with the **maxilla** can be seen here. Behind the maxilla is the

lacrimal bone which houses the nasolacrimal canal, a duct that drains tears from the eye into the nose. The **mandible** articulates with the rest of the skull at the **mandibular condyle**. A depression in front of the condyle is the **mandibular notch** and the anterior section of bone in front of the notch is the **coronoid process**. Label the major features of the skull seen in lateral view and color each bone a different color.

Details of the mandible can be seen in the isolated bone. In addition to the features of the mandible listed above, find the **mandibular foramen** and the **mental foramen** of the mandible. These are holes for the passage of nerves and blood vessels. The main portion of the mandible is the **body** and the upright part is the **ramus**. The **angle** is the posterior junction of these two parts. The teeth are located in alveoli and the small segments of bone between the teeth are the alveolar processes. Label the features of the mandible.

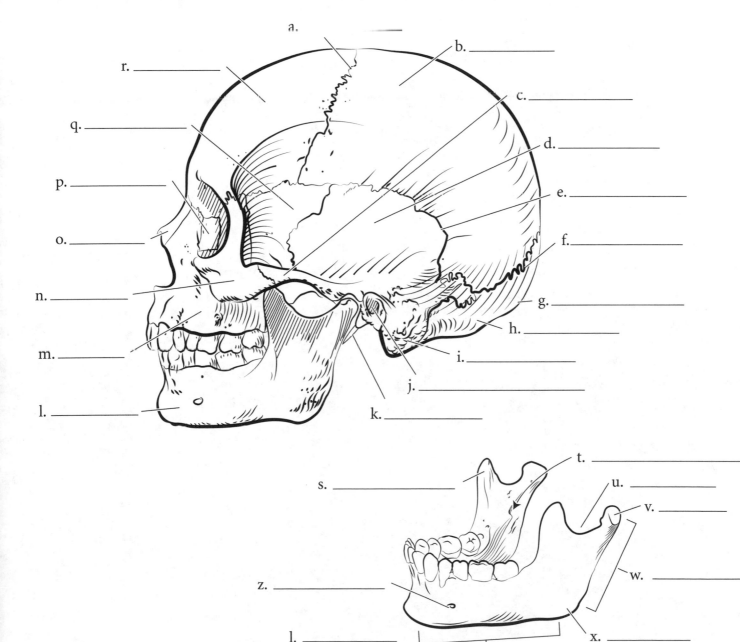

Answer Key: a. Coronal suture, b. Parietal bones, c. Zygomatic process, d. Temporal bone, e. Squamous suture, f. Lambdoid suture, g. External occipital protuberance, h. Occipital bone, i. Mastoid process, j. External acoustic meatus, k. Styloid process, l. Mandible, m. Maxilla, n. Zygomatic bone, o. Nasal bone, p. Lacrimal bone, q. Sphenoid bone, r. Frontal bone, s. Coronoid process, t. Mandibular foramen, u. Mandibular notch, v. Mandibular condyle, w. Ramus, x. Angle, y. Body, z. Mental foramen

SKULL—TOP AND BOTTOM VIEWS

The superior aspect of the skull consists of few bones and few sutures. The **frontal bone** is the most anterior bone with the **parietal bones** directly posterior to it. The **coronal suture** separates the two and the **sagittal suture** separates the parietal bones. The **lambdoid suture** separates the parietal bone from the **occipital bone**. Label the bones and sutures and color the bones in the illustrations.

The inferior aspect of the skull is more complex than the superior view. In the inferior view the mandible has been removed so some of the underlying structures can be seen. The large opening in the occipital bone is the **foramen magnum**. The two bumps lateral to the foramen magnum are the **occipital condyles** and the raised bump at the posterior part of the skull is the **external occipital protuberance**. The more anterior and lateral bone to the occipital bone is the temporal bone. The **jugular foramen** is located between the occipital and temporal bone. Another opening nearby is the **carotid canal**. Lateral to this is the **styloid process**, an attachment point for muscles. Lateral to this is a depression called the **mandibular fossa**. It is here that the mandible articulates with the temporal bone. The **sphenoid bone** spans the skull and the major features seen from the inferior view are the **greater wing**, and the **lateral** and **medial pterygoid plates**. The hard palate is made of the **palatine process of the maxilla** and the **palatine bones**. The bone that opens into the nasal cavity is the **vomer**. Label and color these features of the skull.

Answer Key: a. Frontal bone, b. Coronal suture, c. Parietal bones, d. Sagittal suture, e. Lambdoid suture, f. Occipital bone, g. Palatine process of the maxilla, h. Palatine bone, i. Vomer, j. Greater wing, k. Lateral pterygoid plate, l. Medial pterygoid plate, m. Mandibular fossa, n. Styloid process, o. Carotid canal, p. Jugular foramen, q. Occipital condyles, r. Foramen magnum, s. External occipital protuberance

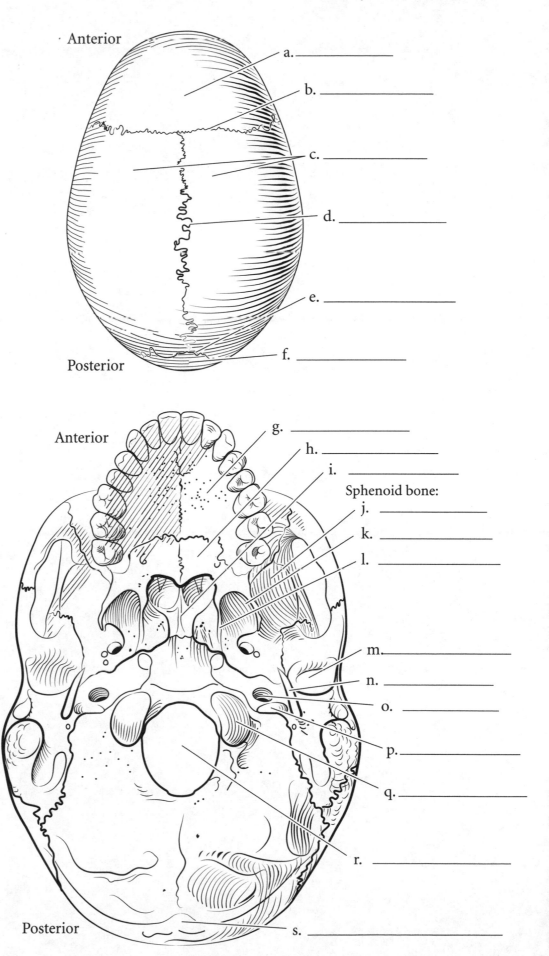

Anterior

a. _____
b. _____
c. _____
d. _____
e. _____
f. _____

Posterior

Anterior

g. _____
h. _____
i. _____
Sphenoid bone:
j. _____
k. _____
l. _____
m. _____
n. _____
o. _____
p. _____
q. _____
r. _____

Posterior

s. _____

MIDSAGITTAL SECTION OF THE SKULL

Several features of the skull can be seen when it is sectioned in the midsagittal plane. Locate the major bones of the skull and the features seen in this section. The nasal septum consists of two bony structures, the **perpendicular plate of the ethmoid bone** and the **vomer**. The **crista galli** extends superiorly from the **cribriform plate** of the ethmoid bone. The junction of the **maxilla** and the **palatine bone** that make up the hard palate can be seen from this view as well. The **frontal sinus** and the **sphenoid sinus** are two cavities seen here. Label the bones and the major features of the midsagittal section of the skull using the terms provided. Color the bones different colors and shade the sinuses in a darker shade of the color used for the specific bones that hold the sinuses.

Frontal bone	Parietal bone	Occipital bone
Temporal bone	Sphenoid bone	Ethmoid bone
Maxilla	Mandible	Internal acoustic meatus
Styloid process	Sella turcica	Cribriform plate of the ethmoid
Nasal bone	Palatine bone	Perpendicular plate of the ethmoid
Vomer	Crista galli	Frontal sinus
Sphenoid sinus		

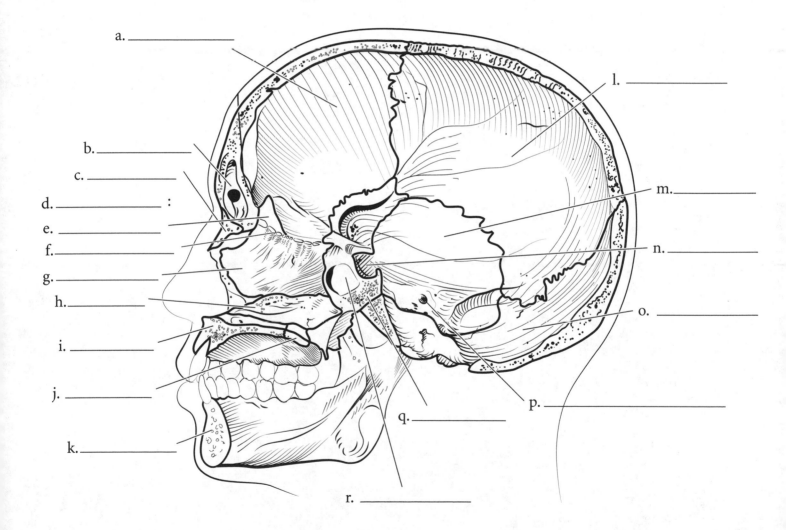

Answer Key: a. Frontal bone, b. Frontal sinus, c. Nasal bone, d. Ethmoid bone, e. Crista galli, f. Cribriform plate of the ethmoid, g. Perpendicular plate of the ethmoid, h. Vomer, i. Maxilla, j. Palatine bone, k. Mandible, l. Parietal bone, m. Temporal bone, n. Sella turcica, o. Occipital bone, p. Internal acoustic meatus, q. Sphenoid bone, r. Sphenoid sinus

SPHENOID, TEMPORAL, AND ETHMOID BONES

A few bones of the skull are frequently studied as separate bones. The sphenoid bone has a superficial resemblance to a bat or butterfly. There are the **lesser wings**, the **greater wings**, and the **pterygoid plates**, all of which resemble wings. The **dorsum sellae** is the posterior part of the **sella turcica** (a depression that holds the pituitary gland). Locate the **foramen rotundum** and the **foramen ovale** on the sphenoid bone. These holes enclose parts of the trigeminal nerve.

The temporal bone has a flat **squamous portion** and a denser petrous portion. The section of the temporal bone that connects to the zygomatic bone is the **zygomatic process**. There are two significant canals or meatuses for hearing. These are the **external acoustic meatus** and the internal acoustic meatus. The **mastoid process** is a large bump that can be palpated directly posterior to the ear. The **styloid process** anchors a number of small muscles.

The ethmoid bone is located just posterior to the nose and is best seen isolated from the rest of the skull bones. The cribriform plate that has small holes called olfactory foramina in it. Locate the **crista galli** and the **perpendicular plate**. The ethmoid has four curved structures lateral to the perpendicular plate. These are the two **superior nasal conchae** and the two **middle nasal conchae**. The **ethmoid sinuses** are numerous small holes in the bone. Locate the structures of these skull bones. Label the illustration and color in the features of the bones.

Answer Key:

(Sphenoid features), a. Sella turcica, b. Lesser wing, c. Foramen rotundum, d. Foramen ovale, e. Dorsum sellae, f. Greater wing

(Temporal features), g. Squamous portion, h. Zygomatic process, i. External acoustic meatus, j. Styloid process, k. Mastoid process

(Ethmoid features), l. Crista galli, m. Middle nasal concha, n. Perpendicular plate, o. Superior nasal concha

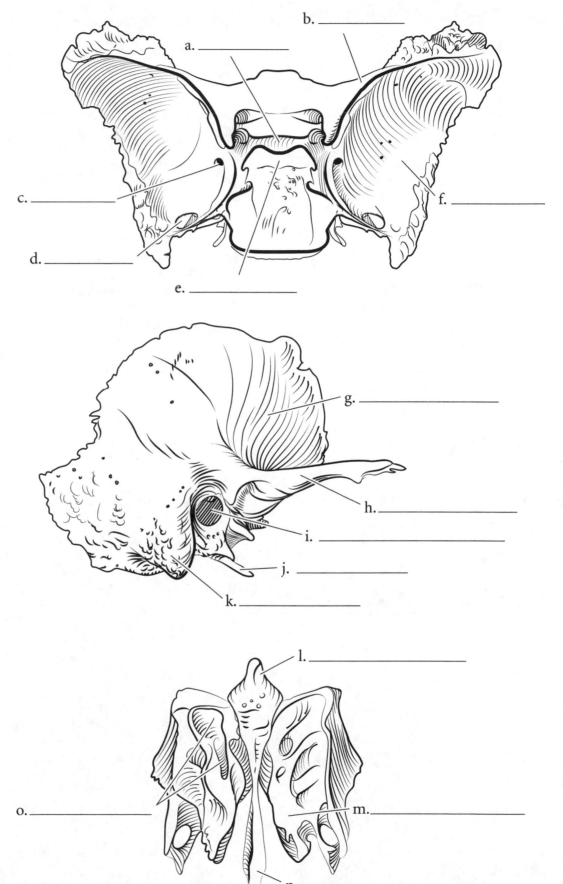

VERTEBRAL COLUMN

We are unique as animals because of our upright posture. The vertical position of the spine is reflected in the increase in size of the vertebra from superior to inferior. The vertebral column is divided into five major regions. There are 7 **cervical vertebrae** that occur in the neck while the 12 **thoracic vertebrae** have ribs attached to them. The 5 **lumbar vertebrae** are found in the lower back and the **sacrum** consists of 5 fused **sacral vertebrae**. The **coccyx** is the terminal portion of the vertebral column consisting of 4 **coccygeal vertebrae**. The vertebral column in the adult has curves. The uppermost is the **cervical curvature** and the lower ones are the **thoracic, lumbar,** and **pelvic curvatures**. Label the illustration with the regions and the curvatures and color in the regions with different colors. Color in the curved arrows for the curvatures.

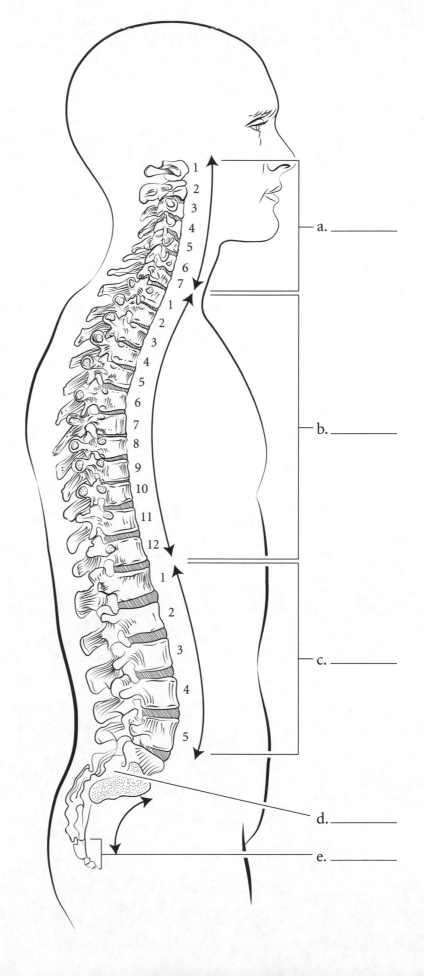

a. _____

b. _____

c. _____

d. _____

e. _____

Answer Key: a. Cervical vertebrae (cervical curvature), b. Thoracic vertebrae (thoracic curvature), c. Lumbar vertebrae (lumbar curvature), d. Sacrum (pelvic curvature), e. Coccyx

ATLAS

The **atlas** is the first cervical vertebra. It is unique among the vertebrae because it has no body. Label the **vertebral foramen**, **superior articular facet**, the **transverse foramen**, and the **lateral masses**.

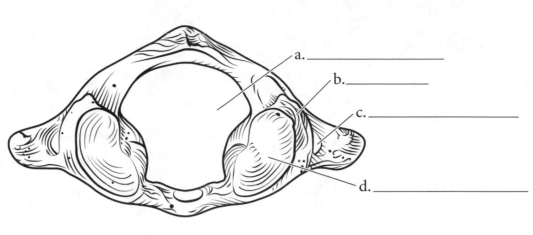

a._____
b._____
c._____
d._____

AXIS

The **axis** is the second cervical vertebra and it has a **body** with a projection that arises from the body known as the **odontoid process** or **dens**. Label the axis including the **superior articular facets**, the **transverse foramen**, the **spinous process**, and the **vertebral foramen**. Color these features in.

e._____
a._____
f._____
c._____
d._____
g._____

ATLAS AND AXIS

Here are the **atlas** and **axis** together. Color the two bones separate colors.

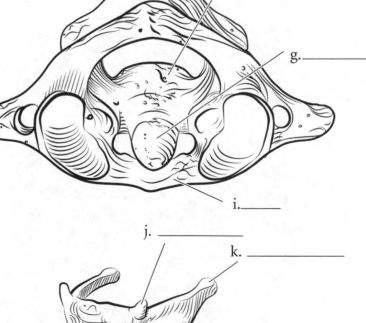

h._____
g._____
i._____

HYOID

The hyoid bone is a floating bone, which means that it has no hard attachments to other bones. The main part of the hyoid is the **body** and the two horns that arise from the hyoid are the **greater cornua** and the **lesser cornua**. Label these parts of the bone and color them in separate colors.

j._____
k._____
l._____

Answer Key: a. Vertebral foramen, b. Lateral masses, c. Transverse foramen, d. Superior articular facet, e. Spinous process, f. Body, g. Odontoid process (dens), h. Axis, i. Atlas, j. Lesser cornua, k. Greater cornua, l. Body

CERVICAL, THORACIC, AND LUMBAR VERTEBRAE

Features common to vertebrae

The opening where the spinal cord passes through the vertebra is known as the **vertebral foramen**. The **body** of the vertebra is the weight-bearing part of the vertebra and the **spinous process** is the part that extends posteriorly. This process is an extension from the **vertebral arch** that curves from the body enclosing the vertebral foramen. This arch is composed of the two **pedicles** and the two **laminae**. The **superior articular process** and the **superior articular facet** (the flat surface on the process) are the parts that join with the vertebra above. The **inferior articular process** and the **inferior articular facet** are the parts of the vertebra that join with the vertebra below.

Typical cervical vertebrae superior and lateral view

Cervical vertebrae are distinct from all other vertebra by having two **transverse foramina**. These house blood vessels. Another characteristic of the cervical vertebrae is that several of them have a **bifid spinous process**

Typical thoracic vertebrae superior and lateral view

The thoracic vertebrae typically have longer **spinous processes** than cervical vertebrae and many of them point in an inferior direction. The **body** is larger in thoracic vertebrae, and they are the only bones with **costal facets** that are attachment points for the heads of ribs. The **transverse processes** can be seen along with the **transverse costal facets**.

Typical lumbar vertebrae superior and lateral view

The lumbar vertebrae have larger bodies because they support more weight. The **spinous process** is shorter and more horizontal in lumbar vertebrae than in thoracic vertebrae. There are no costal facets and no transverse foramina. Label the parts of the vertebrae illustrated and color them in.

Answer Key: a. Bifid spinous process, b. Spinous process, c. Vertebral foramen, d. Lamina, e. Pedicle, f. Superior articular process, g. Transverse process, h. Body, i. Inferior articular process, j. Transverse foramen, k. Superior costal facet, l. Inferior costal facet

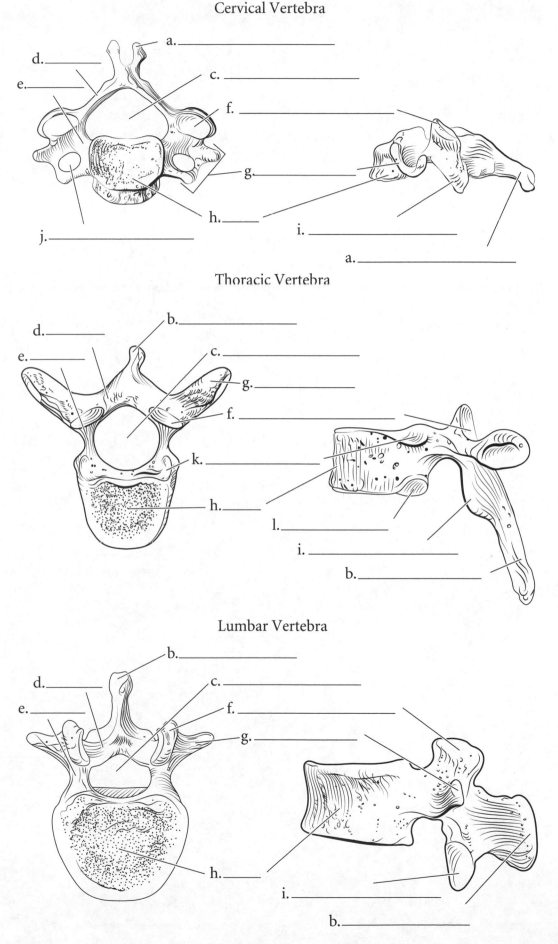

Cervical Vertebra

Thoracic Vertebra

Lumbar Vertebra

SACRUM AND COCCYX

Sacrum and coccyx, anterior view

The terminal portion of the vertebral column consists of two structures that are fused bones. The **sacrum** is 5 fused vertebrae and the **coccyx** is 3–5 fused vertebrae. The top rim of the sacrum is the **sacral promontory** and the wing-like expansion where the ilium attaches is the **ala**. The area where the vertebrae join are the **transverse lines**. The holes running down each side are the **anterior sacral foramina**. At the top of the sacrum are the **superior articular processes** and they attach to the lumbar vertebra. Label and color the parts of the sacrum and the coccyx.

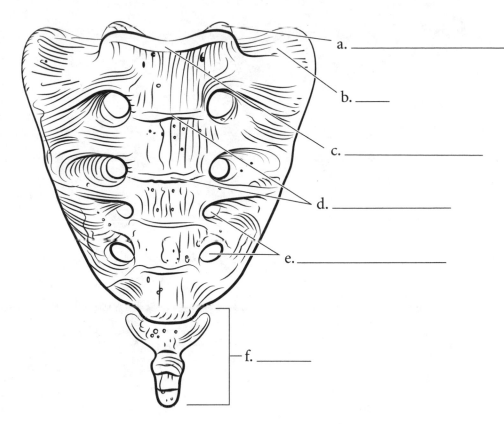

a. _____

b. _____

c. _____

d. _____

e. _____

f. _____

Sacrum and coccyx, posterior view

From the posterior view the **median sacral crest** is the fused remains of the spinous processes of the vertebrae. The **posterior sacral foramina** are on each side of the crest and the **lateral sacral crests** are lateral to the foramina. The **superior articular processes** can be seen from this view and also the **auricular surface** which forms part of the sacroiliac joint. Label the features of the sacrum and the coccyx and color them in.

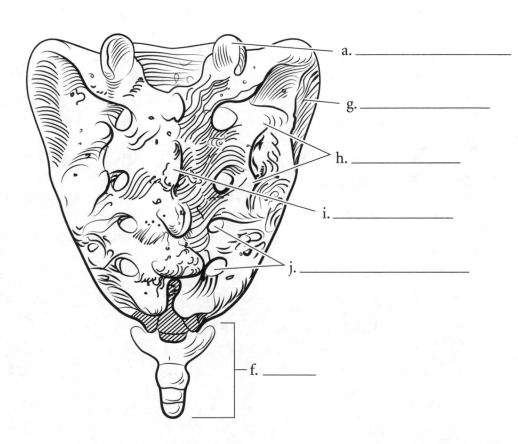

a. _____

g. _____

h. _____

i. _____

j. _____

f. _____

Answer Key: a. Superior articular process, b. Ala, c. Sacral promontory, d. Transverse lines, e. Anterior sacral foramina, f. Coccyx, g. Auricular surface, h. Lateral sacral crest, i. Median sacral crest, j. Posterior sacral foramina

STERNUM / RIBS / HYOID

The **sternum** is commonly known as the breastbone and is divided into three areas, the upper **manubrium** with the **suprasternal notch** and the **clavicular notches**, the **body** with the **costal notches** (where the ribs attach), and the **xiphoid process**. Between the manubrium and the body is the **sternal angle**. Label these features on the illustration and color the three major areas of the sternum different colors.

If you select a rib as a representative bone for all of the ribs, you will find the terminal portion of the rib is expanded in a **head**. The constricted region below that is the **neck**. The **tubercle** of the rib is a bump that attaches to the transverse process of the vertebra. The bend in the rib is known as the **angle** and the depressed area of the rib where nerves and blood vessels are found is the **costal groove**. Color in the individual parts of a rib after you label the figure and color the rib as it joins with a vertebra.

a. _____
b. _____
c. _____
d. _____
e. _____
f. _____
g. _____

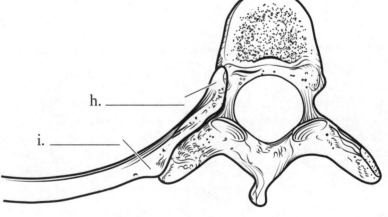

h. _____
i. _____

h. _____
j. _____
k. _____
i. _____
l. _____

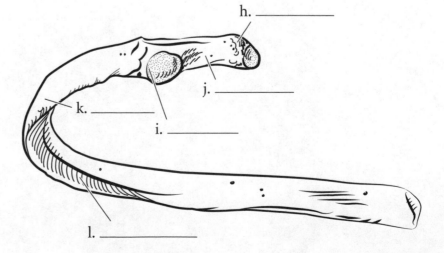

Answer Key: a. Suprasternal notch, b. Clavicular notch, c. Manubrium, d. Sternal angle, e. Costal notches, f. Body, g. Xiphoid process, h. Head, i. Tubercle, j. Neck, k. Angle of rib, l. Costal groove

APPENDICULAR SKELETON—PECTORAL GIRDLE AND UPPER EXTREMITY

The pectoral girdle is made of the **clavicles** and the **scapulae**. The upper extremity consists of the **humerus** of the arm, the **radius** and **ulna** of the forearm, and the **carpals**, **metacarpals**, and **phalanges** of the hand. Locate these major regions of the upper extremity and label them on the diagram. Color these areas in different colors on the illustration.

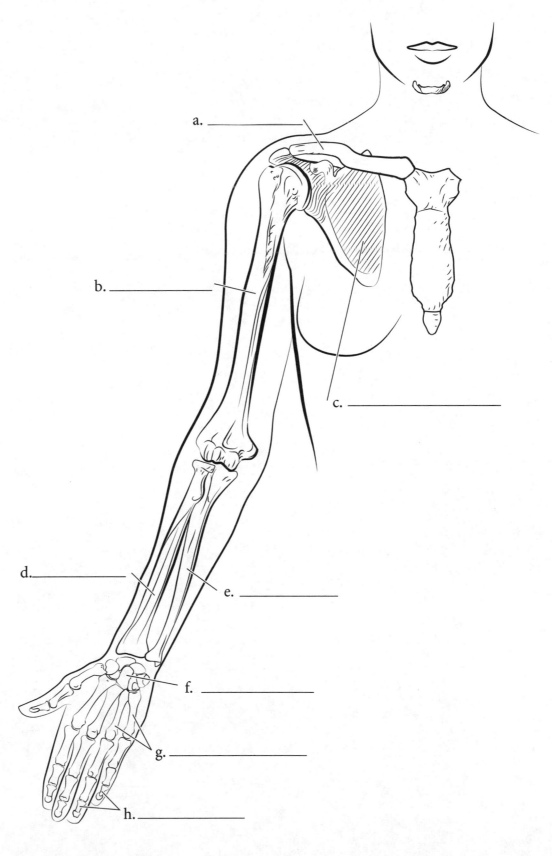

a. _____

b. _____

c. _____

d. _____

e. _____

f. _____

g. _____

h. _____

Answer Key: a. Clavicle, b. Humerus, c. Scapula, d. Radius, e. Ulna, f. Carpals, g. Metacarpals, h. Phalanges

SCAPULA

The pectoral girdle consists of the scapulae and the clavicles. Each scapula is a triangular bone and the three edges are known as the **superior border**, the **lateral border**, and the **medial border**. The **scapular spine** is on the posterior surface and it expands into a terminal process known as the **acromion process**. Above the spine is the **supraspinous fossa**. Below the spine is the **infraspinous fossa** and on the anterior side of the scapula is the **subscapular fossa** and the **coracoid process**. The **inferior angle** of the scapula is at the junction of the medial and lateral borders. Inferior to the acromion process is the **glenoid fossa**. This is a depression where the head of the humerus articulates with the scapula. Label the various features of the scapula and color in the regions of the bone with different colors. Locate as many of the features from the various angles presented.

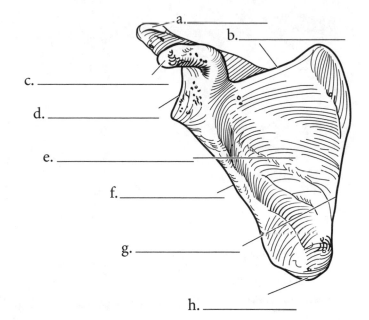

a. _____
b. _____
c. _____
d. _____
e. _____
f. _____
g. _____
h. _____

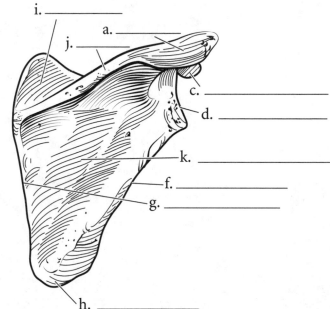

i. _____
a. _____
j. _____
c. _____
d. _____
k. _____
f. _____
g. _____
h. _____

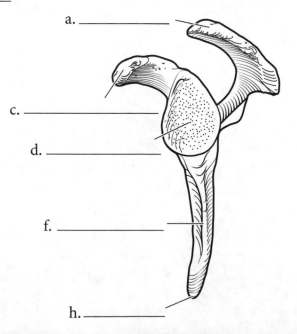

a. _____
c. _____
d. _____
f. _____
h. _____

Answer Key: a. Acromion process,
b. Superior border, c. Coracoid process,
d. Glenoid fossa, e. Subscapular fossa,
f. Lateral border, g. Medial border,
h. Inferior angle, i. Supraspinous fossa,
j. Scapular spine, k. Infraspinous fossa

CLAVICLE

The clavicle is a thin bone that stabilizes the shoulder joint in a lateral position. It has a blunt end that articulates with the sternum (the **sternal end**) and a flattened end that joins with the acromion process of the

scapula. This is called the **acromial end**. A small bump on the inferior part of the clavicle has a ligament that attaches to the coracoid process of the scapula. This bump is called the **conoid tubercle**. Label the clavicle and color the ends and the conoid tubercle.

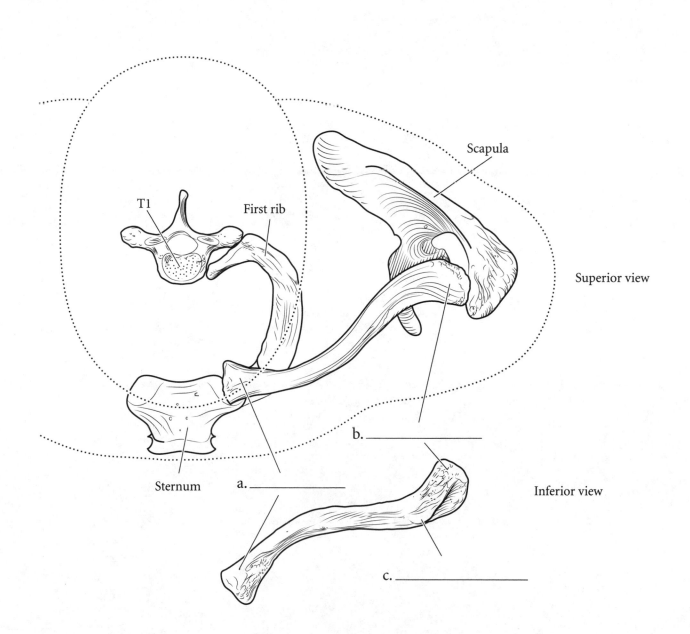

Answer Key: a. Sternal end, b. Acromial end, c. Conoid tubercle

HUMERUS

The humerus has a proximal **head** that fits into the glenoid fossa of the scapula. Just at the edge of the head is a rim known as the **anatomical neck**. Below this neck are the **greater** and **lesser tubercle** and the depression between the two is the **intertubercular groove**. Below these is the **surgical neck** of the humerus. The deltoid muscle attaches to the humerus at the **deltoid tuberosity** and the two expanded wing-like processes at the distal end of the humerus are the **supracondylar ridges**. Inferior to these are the **medial** and **lateral epicondyles** and at the articulating ends of the humerus are the lateral **capitulum** and the medial **trochlea**. The depression on the anterior surface of the humerus into which the ulna fits is called the **coronoid fossa** and the posterior depression where the elbow locks into the humerus is called the **olecranon fossa**. Label the figure and color in the specific parts of the illustration.

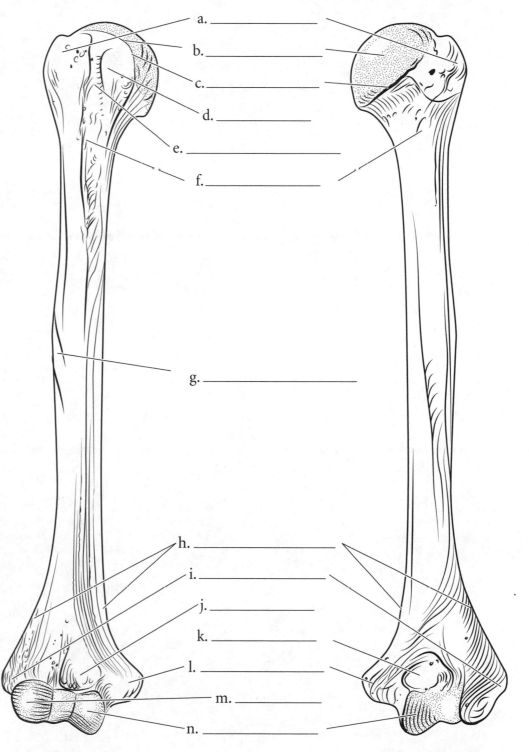

a. _____
b. _____
c. _____
d. _____
e. _____
f. _____

g. _____

h. _____
i. _____
j. _____
k. _____
l. _____
m. _____
n. _____

Anterior View   Posterior View

Answer Key: a. Greater tubercle, b. Head, c. Anatomical neck, d. Lesser tubercle, e. Intertubercular groove, f. Surgical neck, g. Deltoid tuberosity, h. Supracondylar ridges, i. Lateral epicondyle, j. Coronoid fossa, k. Olecranon fossa, l. Medial epicondyle, m. Capitulum, n. Trochlea

FOREARM BONES

The radius has a circular **head**, a **radial tuberosity** on the shaft (where the biceps brachii muscle attaches), and a distal **styloid process**. At the distal end of the radius is a depression where the ulna joins with the radius. This is known as the **ulnar notch** of the radius.

The ulna has a proximal **olecranon process**, a **coronoid process**, and the **trochlear notch** between the two. Just distal to the coronoid process of the ulna is the **tuberosity of the ulna**, a projection where muscles attach. The **head** of the ulna is distal and it also has a **styloid process**. At the proximal portion of the ulna is a depression where the head of the radius articulates with the ulna. This depression is known as the **radial notch** of the ulna.

When the two bones are joined you can see where each fits into the other. On the edge of each bone is the **interosseus margin**. This is a ridge where the interosseus membrane connects the bones.

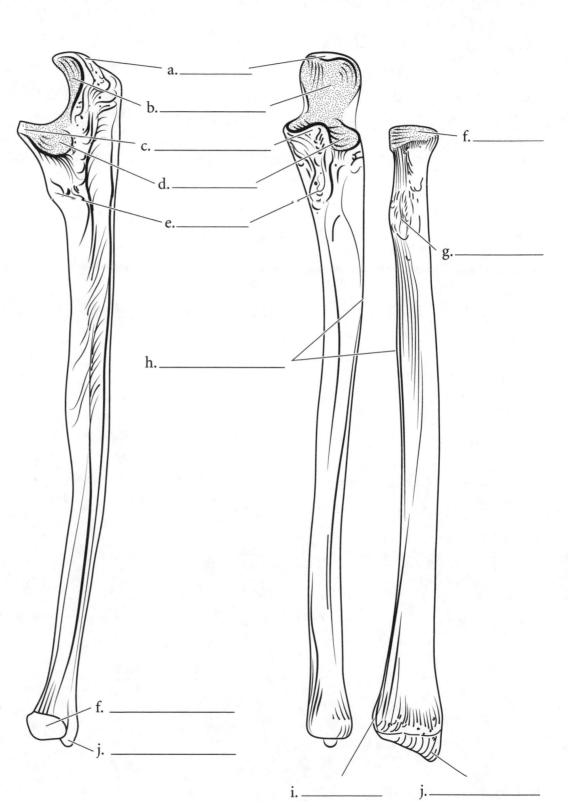

a. _____
b. _____
c. _____
d. _____
e. _____
f. _____
g. _____
h. _____
f. _____
j. _____
i. _____
j. _____

Answer Key: a. Olecranon process, b. Trochlear notch, c. Coronoid process, d. Radial notch, e. Tuberosity of the ulna, f. Head, g. Radial tuberosity, h. Interosseus margin, i. Ulnar notch, j. Styloid process

HAND BONES

The hand consists of 27 bones divided into three groups: the **carpals**, the **metacarpals**, and the **phalanges**. The thumb is known as the **pollex** and is listed as the first digit of the hand. The index finger is the second digit and the fingers are listed sequentially with the little finger being the fifth digit. The bones of the fingers are known as **phalanges** and they are named according to what digit they belong and as being proximal, middle or distal. Therefore the bone of tip of the little finger is the distal phalanx of the fifth digit while the bone in the place where you would normally wear a wedding ring is the proximal phalanx of the fourth digit. Each phalanx has a proximal base, a shaft, and a distal head. The **metacarpals** are the bones of the palm of the hand. Each metacarpal also has a proximal base, a shaft, and a distal head. There are five metacarpals and they are named for the phalanges that extend from them. The first metacarpal articulates with the thumb. The carpals are the bones of the wrist. There are eight carpal bones in two rows. The bone under the thumb is the **trapezium**. The one medial to it is the **trapezoid**. The **capitate** is found under the third metacarpal and the **hamate** finishes that row. Proximal to the trapezium is the **scaphoid**, which joins with the radius. The next bone in line is the **lunate**, followed by the **triquetrum**, and finally the little **pisiform** bone. If you memorize the bones in this sequence you can use a mnemonic device to remember them. This mnemonic is *The Tom Cat Has Shaken Loose To Prowl*. The first letter of the mnemonic represents the first letter of the carpal bone. Label the illustration and color all of the phalanges one color. Color the metacarpals another color and color the carpal bones individual colors. As you color the various illustrations of the hand use the same color scheme for the bones.

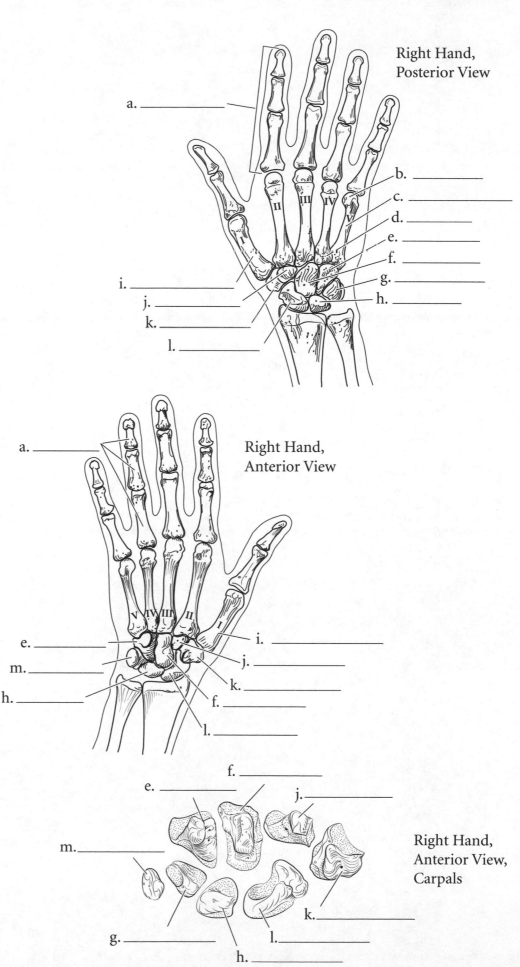

Right Hand, Posterior View

Right Hand, Anterior View

Right Hand, Anterior View, Carpals

Answer Key: a. Phalanges, b. Head, c. Shaft, d. Base, e. Hamate, f. Capitate, g. Triquetrum, h. Lunate, i. Metacarpal, j. Trapezoid, k. Trapezium, l. Scaphoid, m. Pisiform

HIP

The hip bones are known as the os coxae. Each os coxa is a result of the fusion of three bones, the **ilium**, the **ischium**, and the **pubis**. Label and color in these three fused bones using a different color for each area. The two os coxae, when joined together by the **pubic symphysis**, form the pelvis and it can be divided into an upper **false pelvis** and a lower **true pelvis** separated by the pelvic brim. The **anterior superior iliac spine** and the **anterior inferior iliac spine** can be seen from the front. The top ridge of the pelvis is the **iliac crest**. The large, inferior hole is the **obturator foramen** and the depression superior to it is the **acetabulum**. Note the junction of the sacrum and the ilium that forms the **sacroiliac joint**. Label the features of the anterior view and color them in.

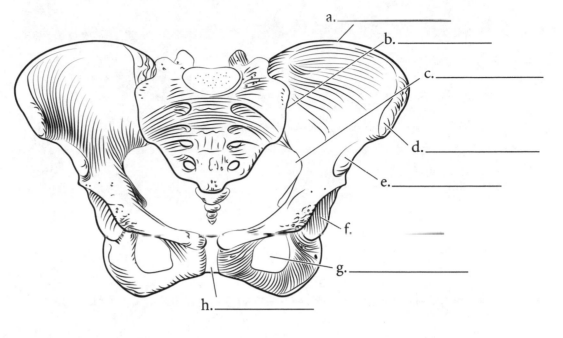

a. _____
b. _____
c. _____
d. _____
e. _____
f.
g. _____
h. _____

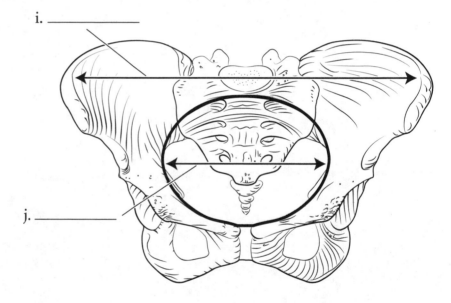

i. _____
j. _____

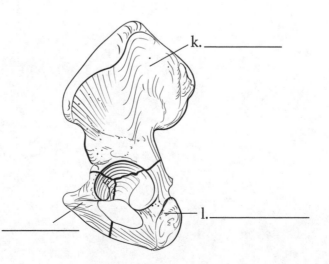

k. _____
l. _____
m. _____

Answer Key: a. Iliac crest, b. Sacroiliac joint, c. Greater sciatic notch, d. Anterior superior iliac spine, e. Anterior inferior iliac spine, f. Acetabulum, g. Obturator foramen, h. Pubic symphysis, i. False pelvis, j. True pelvis, k. Ilium, l. Ischium, m. Pubis

HIP (CONTINUED)

Lateral View

When seen from a lateral view, several features are apparent in the os coxa. Locate the **posterior superior iliac spine** and the **posterior inferior iliac spine** along with the **greater sciatic notch**, the **spine of the ischium**, and the **lesser sciatic notch**. The **ischial tuberosity** is at the posterior, inferior edge of the ischium. Just anterior to the tuberosity is a strip of bone called the **ischial ramus** that attaches to the **inferior pubic ramus**. The body of the pubis is the most anterior part of the pubis and the **superior pubic ramus** is the portion that forms part of the acetabulum. Label and color these features on the illustration.

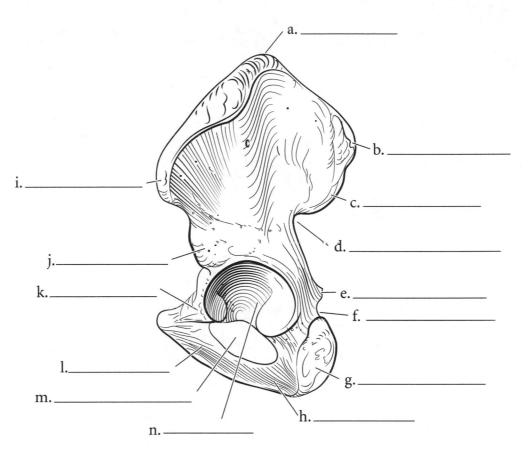

a. _____
b. _____
c. _____
d. _____
e. _____
f. _____
g. _____
h. _____
i. _____
j. _____
k. _____
l. _____
m. _____
n. _____

MALE AND FEMALE PELVIS

Differences can be seen between the male and female pelvis. The **subpubic angle** in males is less than 90 degrees and the female angle is greater than 90 degrees. The ilium in males is more vertical than in a pelvis of a woman who has had children. A further distinction is seen in the side view of a pelvis in which the sciatic notch in the female pelvis has a much wider angle than in males. Color in the upper portion of the ilium.

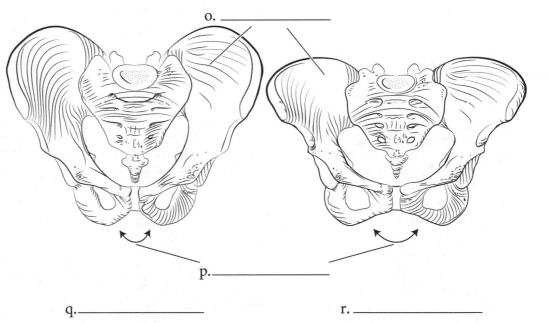

o. _____
p. _____
q. _____
r. _____

Answer Key: a. Iliac crest, b. Posterior superior iliac spine, c. Posterior inferior iliac spine, d. Greater sciatic notch, e. Spine of the ischium, f. Lesser sciatic notch, g. Ischial tuberosity, h. Ischial ramus, i. Anterior superior iliac spine, j. Anterior inferior iliac spine, k. Superior pubic ramus, l. Inferior pubic ramus, m. Obturator foramen, n. Acetabulum, o. Iliac blade, p. Subpubic angle, q. Male (less than ninety degrees), r. Female (more than ninety degrees)

LOWER EXTREMITY—FEMUR/PATELLA

The lower extremity consists of the **femur** of the thigh, the **tibia** and **fibula** of the leg, and the **tarsals**, **metatarsals**, and **phalanges** of the foot. Locate these major regions of the lower extremity and label them on the diagram. Color these areas in different colors on the illustration.

The femur seen from the anterior view shows a proximal **head** and a constricted **neck**. Two large processes are distal to the neck. These are the **greater trochanter** and the **lesser trochanter**. There is a raised section of bone between them called the **intertrochanteric line**. The main part of the bone is the shaft and the **lateral epicondyle** and **medial epicondyle** are the distal expansions of the bone. The posterior view of the femur has additional features such as the **intertrochanteric ridge**, the **linea aspera**, and the **lateral condyle** and the **medial condyle**. The femur is bowed and this can be seen from a lateral view as well as the placement of the **patella**. The **base** of the patella is superior and the **apex** is inferior. Label the features of the femur and patella and color in the various parts.

Answer Key: a. Femur, b. Patella, c. Tibia, d. Fibula, e. Tarsals, f. Metatarsals, g. Phalanges, h. Greater trochanter, i. Head, j. Neck, k. Intertrochanteric line, l. Intertrochanteric ridge, m. Lesser trochanter, n. Linea aspera , o. Lateral epicondyle, p. Lateral condyle, q. Medial epicondyle, r. Medial condyle, s. Base of patella, t. Apex of patella

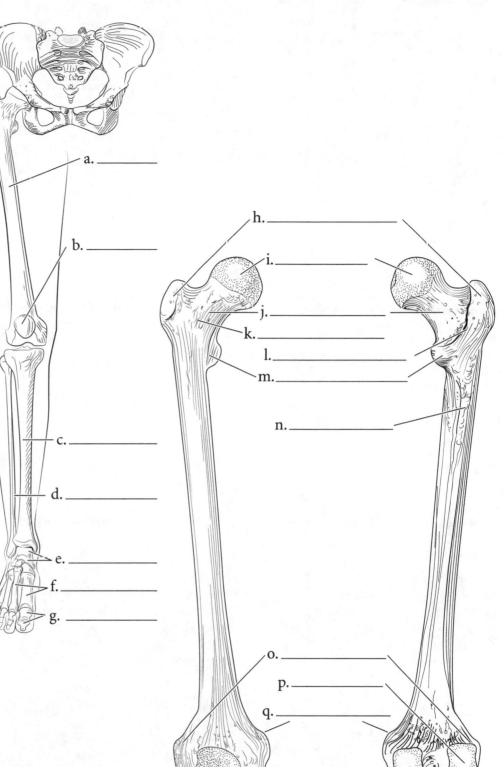

a. _____
b. _____
c. _____
d. _____
e. _____
f. _____
g. _____

h. _____
i. _____
j. _____
k. _____
l. _____
m. _____
n. _____
o. _____
p. _____
q. _____
r. _____
s. _____
t. _____

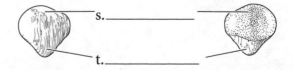

Anterior   Posterior

TIBIA / FIBULA

The **tibia** supports the weight of the body and is the bone that articulates with the femur. The **fibula** is more slender and is a bone to which muscles attach. The top of the tibia is expanded into a triangular shape with the **medial tibial condyle** and **lateral tibial condyle** articulating with the condyles of the femur. The quadriceps femoris muscles attach to the **tibial tuberosity** on the anterior surface of the tibia just below the condyles. The **anterior tibial crest** is a large ridge that runs the length of the bone. At the terminal portion of the tibia is the **medial malleolus**. This process, along with the **lateral malleolus** of the fibula, join with the talus of the foot. The **head** of the fibula is proximal. It is a triangular region with a pointed **apex**. Label the tibia and fibula illustrations and color in the various regions of the bones.

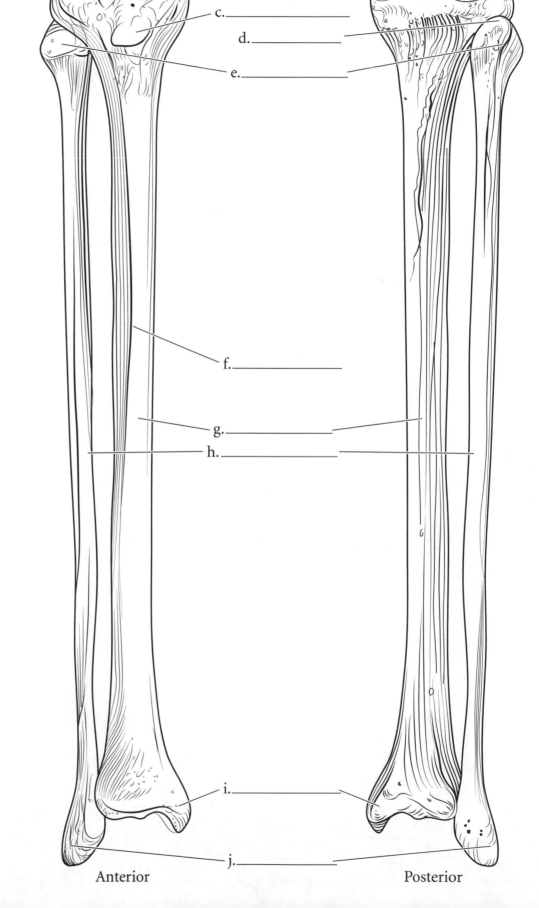

a.
b.
c.
d.
e.

f.

g.

h.

i.

j.

Anterior   Posterior

Answer Key: a. Lateral tibial condyle, b. Medial tibial condyle, c. Tibial tuberosity, d. Apex, e. Head of fibula, f. Anterior tibial crest, g. Shaft of tibia, h. Shaft of fibula, i. Medial malleolus, j. Lateral malleolus

LEFT FOOT

Color in the seven **tarsal** bones using different colors for each bone. The **calcaneus** is the heel bone and takes the major weight of the body during walking. The **talus** connects the foot to the tibia and fibula forming the ankle joint. The **cuneiforms** are so called because they are wedge-shaped bones and they form a natural arch of bone in the foot.

Note that each of the **metatarsals** and each of the **phalanges** has a distal head, a shaft, and a proximal base. Color all of the five metatarsals the same color. The first metatarsal is under the big toe and the fifth is under the smallest toe. Color all of the fourteen phalanges another color. All of the proximal phalanges are given the same letter in the illustration as are the middle and distal phalanges. Write **proximal**, **middle**, or **distal** in the appropriate space next to the toes. The big toe (hallux) has two phalanges while the other toes have three.

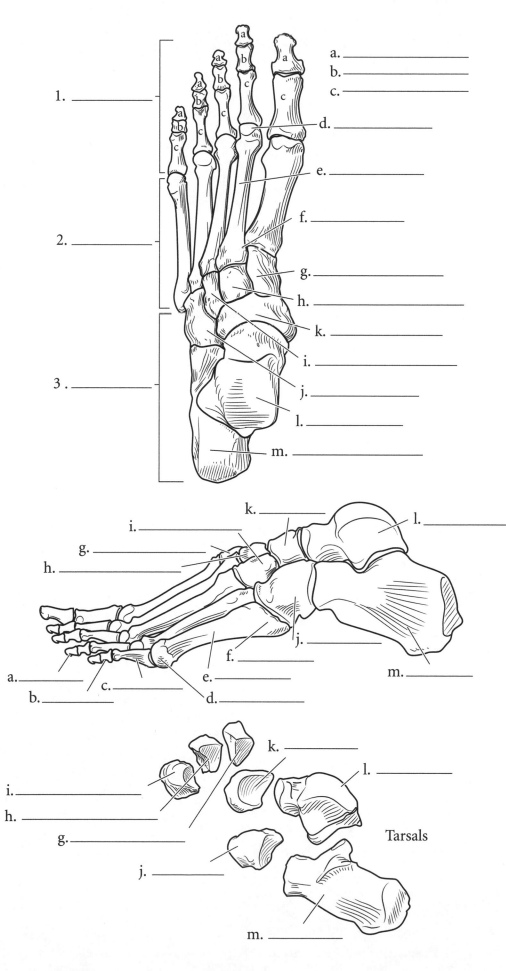

Answer Key:

1. Phalanges
2. Metatarsals
3. Tarsals
a. Distal phalanges,
b. Middle phalanges, c. Proximal phalanges, d. Head, e. Shaft, f. Base,
g. First (medial) cuneiform, h. Second (intermediate) cuneiform,
i. Third (lateral) cuneiform, j. Cuboid, k. Navicular, l. Talus, m. Calcaneus

CLASSIFICATIONS OF ARTICULATIONS

Articulations are the joints that occur between bones. They can be classified either according to movement or by structure. Joints can be immovable (**synarthroses**), semimovable (**amphiarthroses**), or freely movable (**diarthroses**). The composition of joints can be **fibrous**, **cartilaginous**, or **synovial**.

FIBROUS JOINTS

Fibrous joints are held together by collagenous fibers, the same fibers that make up tendons and ligaments. These joints do not have a joint cavity. **Sutures** are immovable fibrous joints of the skull. Color in the suture illustrated on the page. A **gomphosis** is a fibrous joint in which a round peg is held into a socket. Gomphoses are represented by the teeth held into the maxilla or the mandible. Another fibrous joint is the **syndesmosis**. This joint is found between the distal radius and ulna (or tibia and fibula) and is semimovable. Color in the various fibrous joints.

a. _____

b. _____

c. _____

d. _____

e. _____

f. _____

g. _____

h. _____

i. _____

j. _____

k. _____

l. _____

m. _____

n. _____

Answer Key: a. Gomphosis (peg suture), b. Tooth, c. Alveolar socket, d. Gingiva, e. Alveolar ridge, f. Periodontal ligaments, g. Suture, h. Sagittal suture, i. Syndesmosis, j. Tibia, k. Fibula, l. Interosseous membrane, m. Posterior tibiofibular ligament, n. Transverse tibiofibular ligament

CARTILAGINOUS JOINTS

Cartilaginous joints are bones held together by **cartilage** and do not have a joint cavity. If the joint is held together by hyaline cartilage it is known as a **synchondrosis**. If the cartilage is short then the joint is immovable. An example of this kind of joint is an **epiphyseal plate**. If the cartilage is a little longer then the joint is a semimovable joint. This is represented by the **sternal-rib junction**. A cartilaginous joint that is composed of **fibrocartilage** is known as a **symphysis** (**symphyses** plural). These are semimovable joints. Examples of symphyses are the pubic symphysis and intervertebral discs. Color the cartilaginous joints. Use different colors for the hyaline cartilage from the fibrocartilage.

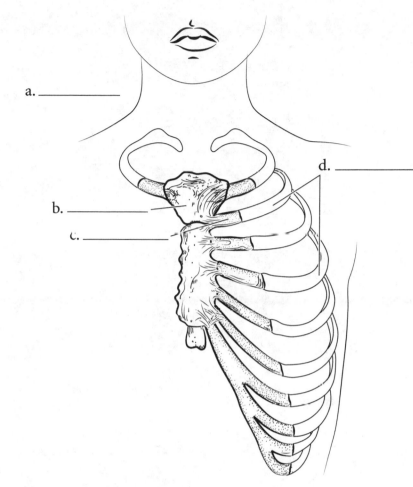

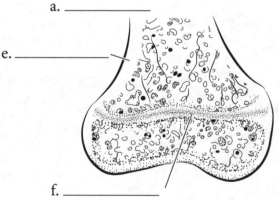

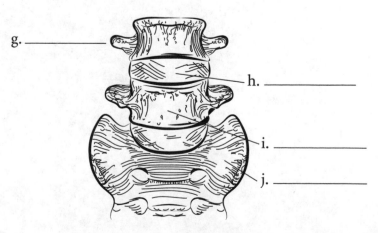

Answer Key: a. Synchondrosis,
b. Sternum, c. Costal cartilage,
d. Ribs, e. Femur, f. Epiphyseal plate,
g. Symphysis, h. Intervertebral disc,
i. Lumbar vertebra, j. Sacrum

SYNOVIAL JOINTS, BURSA, AND TENDON SHEATH

Synovial joints are complex joints that are all freely movable. There are variations with the joints but all synovial joints consist of two **bones** enclosed by a **joint capsule**, **articular cartilages**, **synovial membranes** that secrete **synovial fluid** in the **synovial cavity**. Some synovial joints have fibrocartilage pads in the cavity called **menisci** (**meniscus** singular). Color the synovial joint and pay attention to the general structure of the joint. Color each part of the joint a different color.

MODIFIED SYNOVIAL STRUCTURES—BURSAE AND TENDON SHEATHS

There are structures in the body that consist of synovial membranes and fibrous capsules. These are not synovial joints but are associated with joints. A bursa is one such structure. It is a fluid-filled sac with an internal synovial membrane that cushions tendons as they pass over bones. The bursa occurs between the tendon and the bone. Another structure is a tendon sheath. It also is composed of a synovial membrane and fibrous sheath and it encloses tendons. The sheaths can provide lubrication to the tendon so it does not become irritated as it passes over bones or next to other tendons. Color in the layers of the bursa and the tendon sheaths.

Answer Key: a. Bone, b. Joint capsule, c. Synovial cavity (synovial fluid), d. Meniscus, e. Articular cartilage, f. Synovial membrane, g. Tendon sheath, h. Achilles tendon, i. Bursa, j. Calcaneus

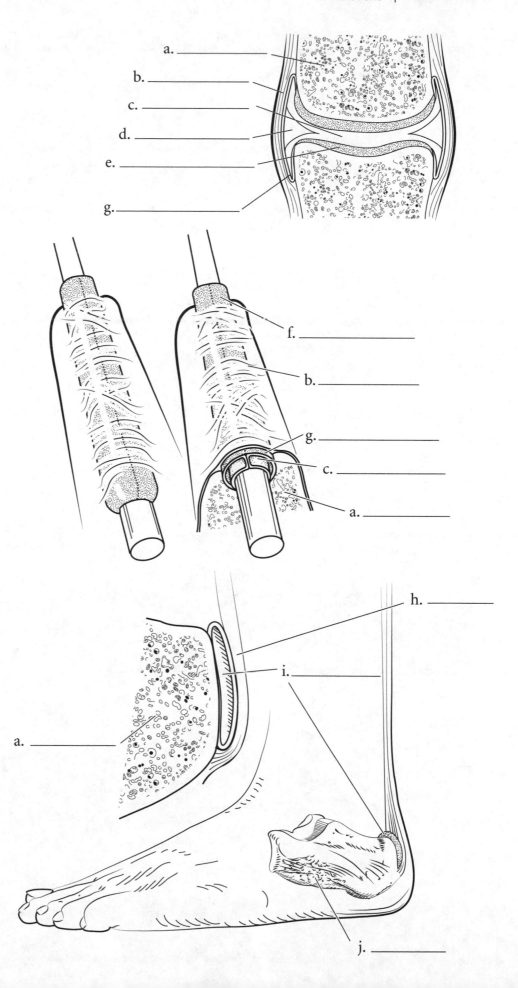

SPECIFIC SYNOVIAL JOINTS

Synovial joints are classified by what kind of motion they have. **Gliding joints** move in one plane like two sheets of glass sliding across one another. **Hinge joints** have angular movement like a door hinge. **Rotating (pivot) joints** move like a wheel of a car around an axle. **Condyloid (ellipsoidal) joints** move like hinges in two directions. In these joints there is a convex surface and a concave surface. **Saddle joints** have two concave surfaces. They allow for greater movement than condyloid joints. **Ball and socket** joints allow for the greatest range of movement and are found in the shoulder and hip. Color the illustrations of these joints.

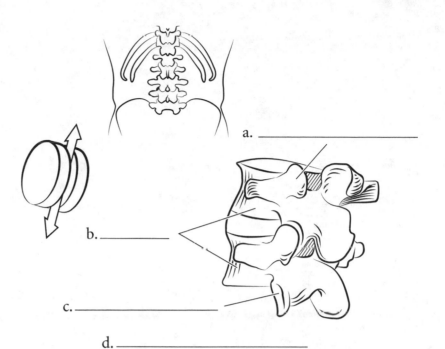

a. _____

b. _____

c. _____

d. _____

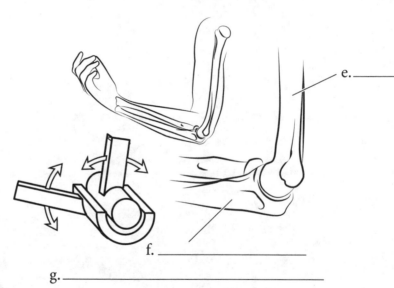

e. _____

f. _____

g. _____

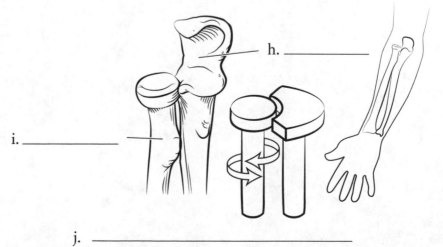

h. _____

i. _____

j. _____

Answer Key: a. Superior articular process, b. Vertebrae, c. Inferior articular process, d. Gliding (plane), e. Humerus, f. Ulna, g. Hinge, h. Ulna, i. Radius, j. Rotating

SPECIFIC SYNOVIAL
JOINTS (CONTINUED)

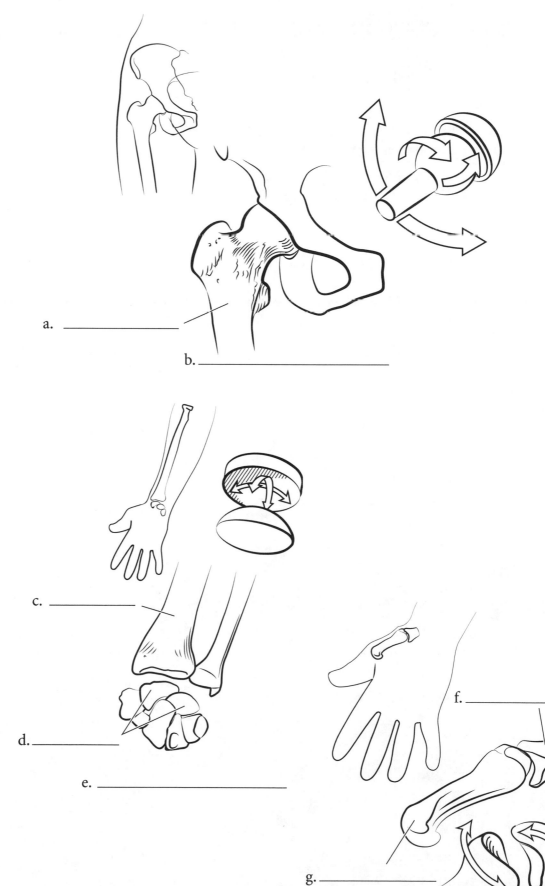

a. _____

b. _____

c. _____

d. _____

e. _____

f. _____

g. _____

h. _____

SPECIFIC JOINTS

TEMPOROMANDIBULAR JOINT

Some joints of the body warrant special attention. The **temporomandibular joint** or **jaw joint** is both a gliding joint and a **hinge joint**. The **condyle** of the mandible articulates with the **mandibular fossa** of the temporal bone. An **articular disc** is found in the joint that decreases the stress on the joint. Ligaments (dense connective tissue that joins bone to bone) connect the mandible to the temporal bone.

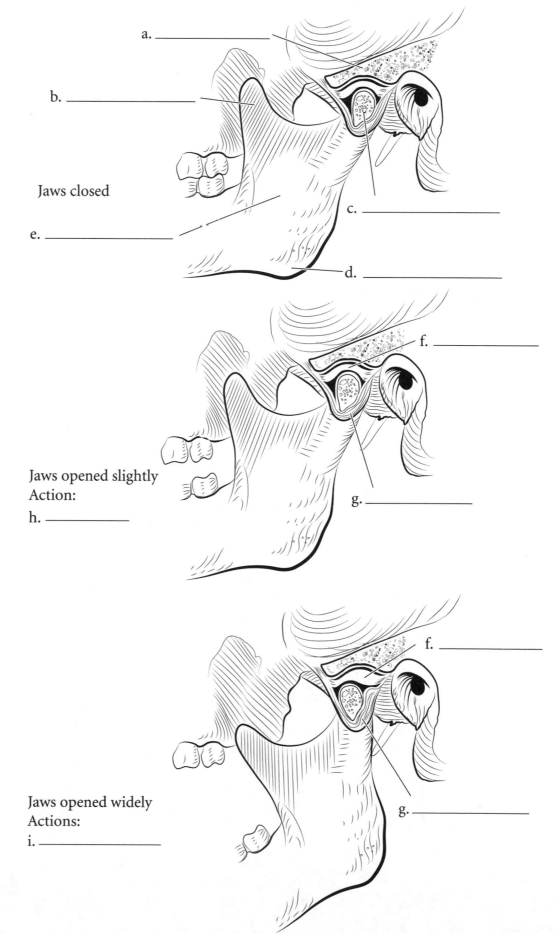

a. _____

b. _____

Jaws closed

c. _____

e. _____

d. _____

f. _____

Jaws opened slightly
Action:
h. _____

g. _____

f. _____

Jaws opened widely
Actions:
i. _____

g. _____

Answer Key: a. Temporal bone, b. Coronoid process, c. Condyloid process (cut), d. Angle of mandible, e. Mandibl,. f. Articular disc, g. Capsule, h. Hinge, i. Hinge and glide

HUMEROSCAPULAR AND ACETABULOFEMORAL JOINTS

The **humeroscapular joint** or shoulder joint is a ball-and-socket joint that connects the **humerus** to the **glenoid fossa** of the scapula. The joint is deepened by the **glenoid labrum** which is a **fibrocartilage** ring. There are numerous ligaments that connect the scapula to the humerus.

Another ball and socket joint is the **acetabulofemoral joint.** It also has an **acetabular labrum** and numerous ligaments that joint the femur to the hip.

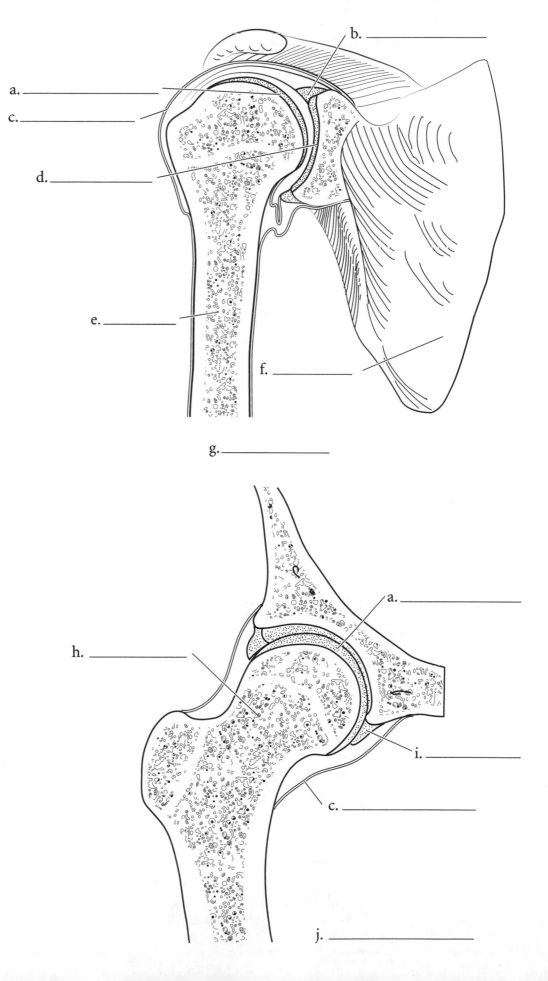

TIBIOFEMORAL JOINT

The **tibiofemoral joint** is special in humans because it is the largest joint in the body and because it is particularly vulnerable to injury. The joint is stabilized by the **patellar tendon**, the **medial** and **lateral collateral ligaments**, the **anterior** and **posterior cruciate ligaments** and the **medial** and **lateral menisci**. Label the structures in the anterior view, with the patella in place and with it reflected, and color them in.

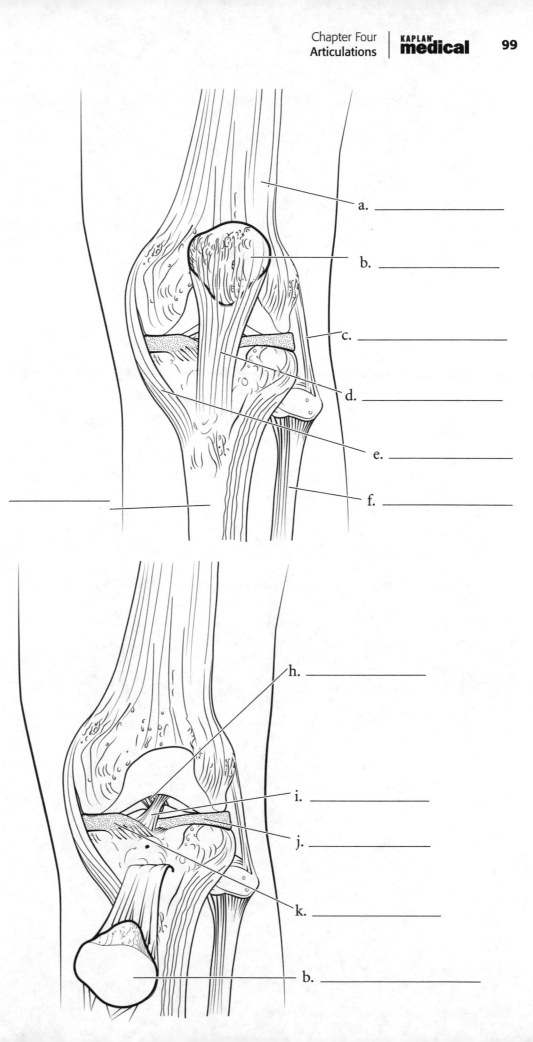

a. _____

b. _____

c. _____

d. _____

e. _____

f. _____

g. _____

h. _____

i. _____

j. _____

k. _____

b. _____

Answer Key: a. Femur, b. Patella,
c. Fibular collateral ligament,
d. Patellar tendon, e. Tibial collateral
ligament, f. Fibula, g. Tibia,
h. Posterior cruciate ligament,
i. Anterior cruciate ligament,
j. Lateral meniscus,
k. Medial meniscus

MOVEMENT AT JOINTS

There is a broad range of motion that occurs at joints. These motions should be referenced with the body in anatomical position. **Flexion** of a joint is a decrease in the joint angle from the body in anatomic position. When the elbow is bent the forearm is flexed. Most flexion takes place in a forward direction. The exception to this is the leg where flexion of the leg results in the bending of the knee. **Extension** of the joint is when the joint is returned to anatomic position. **Hyperextension** is a condition where the joint is extended beyond anatomic position. Looking up at the ceiling is hyperextension of the head.

Abduction occurs when the extremities or head are moved in the coronal plane, laterally from the body. **Adduction** is the return of the limbs to the body.

Rotation is the movement of part of the body in a circular pattern. **Lateral rotation** is the movement of the body in a lateral direction and **medial rotation** is in the opposite direction.

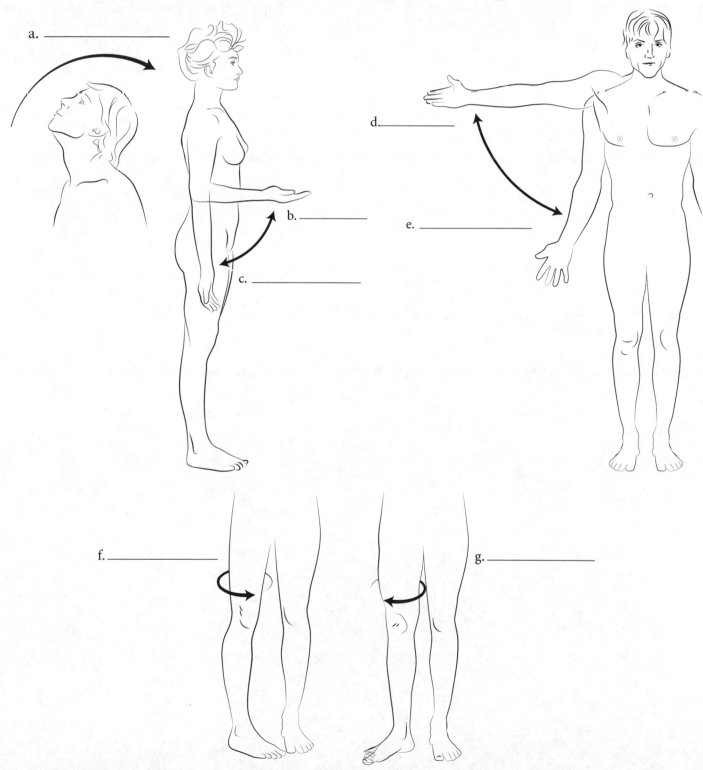

Answer Key: a. Hyperextension of the head, b. Flexion of the forearm, c. Extension of the forearm, d. Abduction of the arm, e. Adduction of the arm, f. Medial rotation of the thigh, g. Lateral rotation of the thigh

OVERVIEW OF THE NERVOUS SYSTEM

The body must react to the external environment and the internal environment and communicate information between regions of the body. This job is primarily the task of the nervous system. Proper response to the external environment is critical for thermal regulation, response to threats, taking advantage of opportunities such as food availability, and a host of other stimuli. Response to the internal environment is important for sensing muscle tension, digestive processes, maintenance of blood pressure, and other functions. Communication is important for coordination of activities such as walking, digestion, and maintenance of blood pressure. The nervous system also integrates information from the environment, relates past information to the present and interprets new experiences. The **brain** and the **spinal cord** make up the **central nervous system**. The nerves of the body make up the **peripheral nervous system**. The peripheral nervous system is divided into the **somatic nervous system** which consists of **spinal nerves** and **peripheral nerves** that innervate the outer regions of the body. It also consists of the **autonomic nervous system**. Label the parts of the nervous system and color them in.

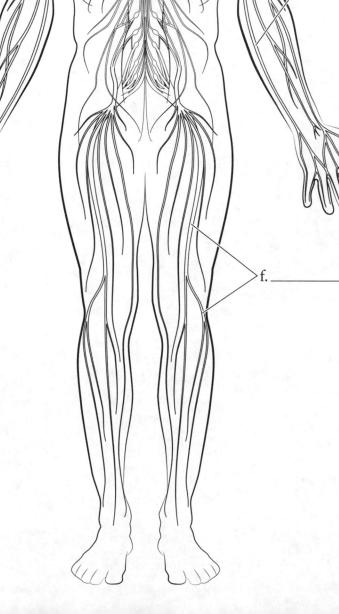

a._____ :

b._____

c._____

d._____ :

e._____

f._____

f._____

NEURON

The nerve cell or **neuron** is the functional cell in the nervous system. Most electrical conduction in the body is due to the transmission of impulses by the neuron. The neuron consists of branched structures called **dendrites**. The main portion of the nerve cell is called the **soma** or **nerve cell body**, and the elongated part of the neuron is the **axon**. Two neurons are connected by gaps called **synapses**. The nerve cell body is the metabolic center of the cell consisting of a nucleus, an endoplasmic reticulum called the **Nissl bodies**, and a region where the axon attaches called the **axon hillock**. Color in the parts of the neuron and label the parts.

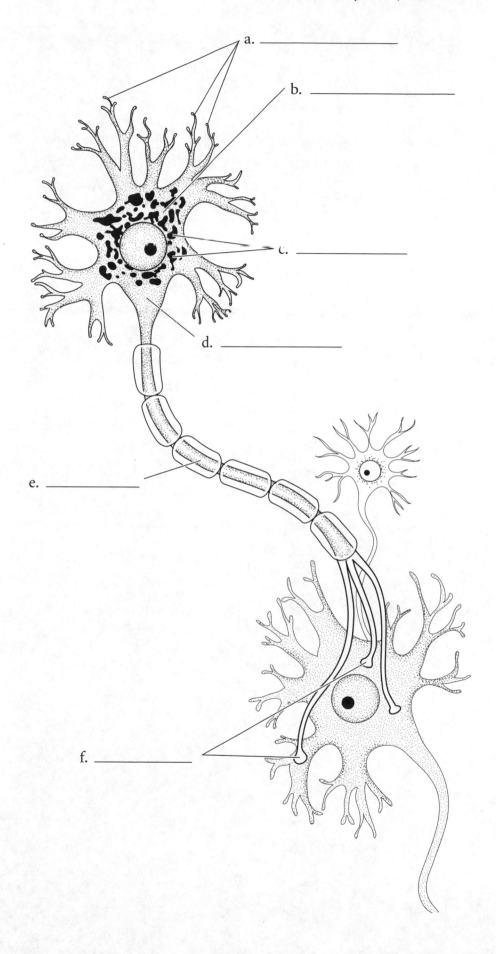

a. _____

b. _____

c. _____

d. _____

e. _____

f. _____

NEUROGLIA

Neuroglia or **glial cells** have many specialized functions in the nervous system. The **neurolemmocyte** or **Schwann cell** is found in the peripheral nervous system. These cells make up the **myelin sheath** that wraps around **axons.**

The other neuroglia are located in the central nervous system. **Astrocytes** are glial cells that, along with the brain capillaries, are found in the blood-brain barrier. They also have a role in transferring nutrients from the capillaries to the deeper regions of the brain. Another glial cell that functions as a barrier is the **ependymal** cell. These cells are located between the CNS and cavities filled with cerebrospinal fluid. **Microglia** are also found in the CNS and their function is one of protection. Microglia respond to invasions of the nervous system and they destroy microbes.

Oligodendrocytes are neuroglia that produce myelination in the CNS. Myelinated nerve fibers comprise white matter. Myelinated fibers conduct impulses faster than unmyelinated fibers. White matter is mostly associated with transmission of neural impulses from one area to another. Color each glial cell a different color and write the name of each cell in the space provided.

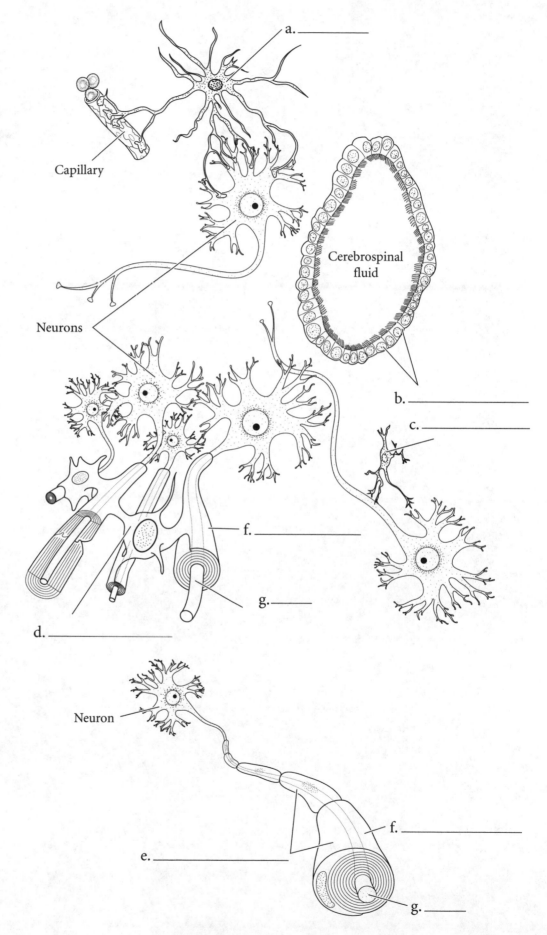

a. _____

Capillary

Cerebrospinal fluid

Neurons

b. _____

c. _____

f. _____

g. _____

d. _____

Neuron

f. _____

e. _____

g. _____

Answer Key: a. Astrocyte,
b. Ependymal cell, c. Microglial cell,
d. Oligodendrocyte,
e. Neurolemmocytes (Schwann cells),
f. Myelin sheath, g. Axon

NEURON SHAPES/SYNAPSE

Neurons come in a few basic shapes. The most common neuron in the CNS is the **multipolar neuron**. It consists of many dendrites and a single axon. **Bipolar neurons** are not very common. They are found in the eye, in the nose, and in the ear and consist of a singular dendrite and an axon. **Pseudounipolar neurons** make up the sensory nerves of the body. They consist of a cluster of dendrites at one end, a long axon leading to the nerve cell body, and another axon leaving the nerve cell body at the same area.

Neurons connect to each other by synapses. The neuron first carrying the information is called the **presynaptic neuron**. This neuron has **synaptic vesicles** that release **neurotransmitters**. The **synaptic cleft** is the space between the neurons and the **postsynaptic neuron** is the receiving neuron. Label the various neurons and their parts as well as the synapse between the neurons.

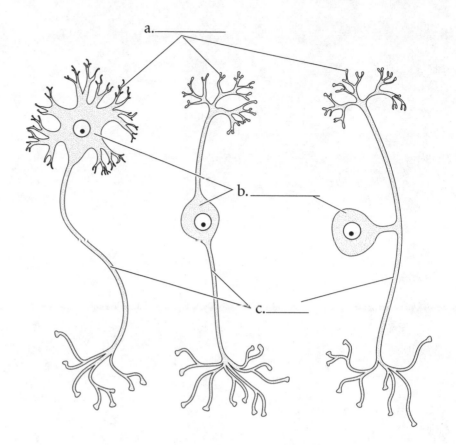

d._____ e._____ f._____

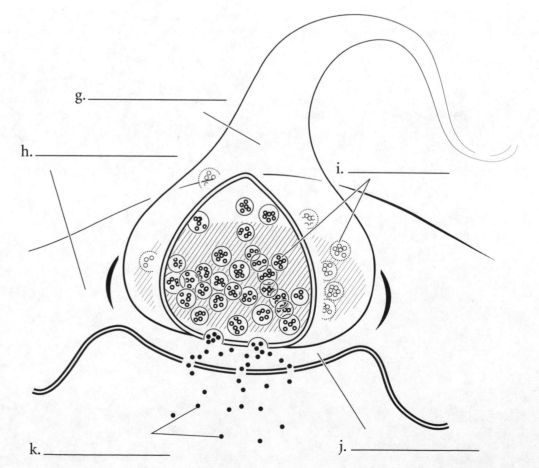

g._____

h._____

i._____

k._____   j._____

Answer Key: a. Dendrites, b. Nerve cell body, c. Axon, d. Multipolar neuron, e. Bipolar neuron, f. Pseudounipolar neuron, g. Presynaptic neuron, h. Postsynaptic neuron, i. Synaptic vesicles, j. Synaptic cleft, k. Neurotransmitter

NEURAL DEVELOPMENT

The nervous system develops early as a neural groove. This groove folds in on itself to become a neural tube as early as four weeks after conception. At about six weeks of age the beginning cerebral hemispheres can be seen as lateral enclosures from the neural tube along with the **developing eye** just posterior to the hemispheres. This embryonic brain is divided into three regions, the **prosencephalon** or forebrain, the **mesencephalon** or midbrain, and the **rhombencephalon** or hindbrain. Label the parts of the embryonic brain and the adult derivatives of that brain and color in the regions.

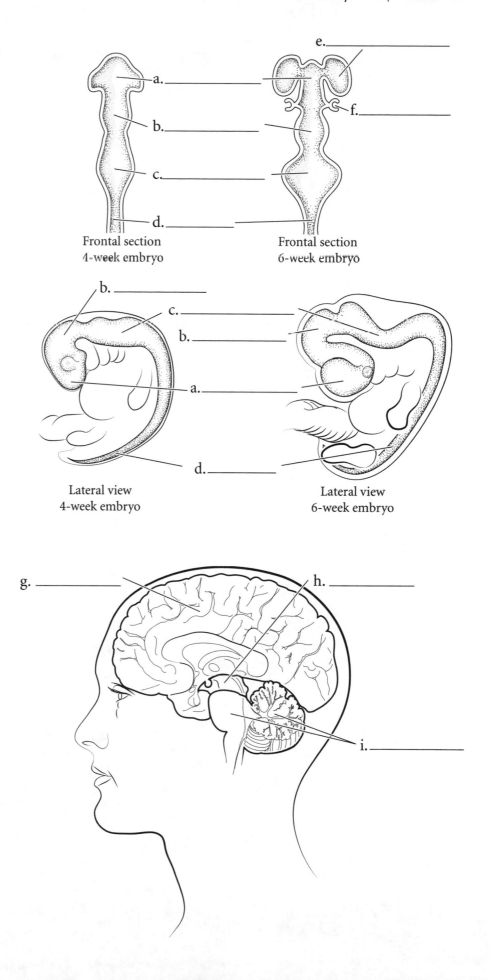

Frontal section
4-week embryo

Frontal section
6-week embryo

Lateral view
4-week embryo

Lateral view
6-week embryo

Answer Key: a. Prosencephalon,
b. Mesencephalon,
c. Rhombencephalon, d. Spinal cord,
e. Cerebral hemisphere, f. Developing
eye, g. Forebrain, h. Midbrain,
i. Hindbrain

LATERAL ASPECT OF THE BRAIN

The most obvious features of a lateral view of the brain are the lobes of the cerebrum and the **cerebellum**. The most anterior lobe is the **frontal lobe**, which is responsible for intellect and abstract reasoning, among other things. The division between the frontal lobe and the **parietal lobe** is the **central sulcus**. Just anterior to the central sulcus is the **precentral gyrus**, an area that sends motor impulses to muscles of the body. Just posterior to the central sulcus is the **postcentral gyrus**. The postcentral gyrus receives sensory information from the body. On the lateral aspect of the brain is the **lateral fissure** and inferior to this is the **temporal lobe** of the brain. Hearing, taste, smell, and the formation of memories all have centers here. The most posterior part of the cerebrum is the **occipital lobe,** which has visual interpretation areas. Label the regions seen in a lateral view of the brain and the spinal cord. Color the precentral and postcentral gyri and then color the lobes of the brain. Shade in the cerebellum as well.

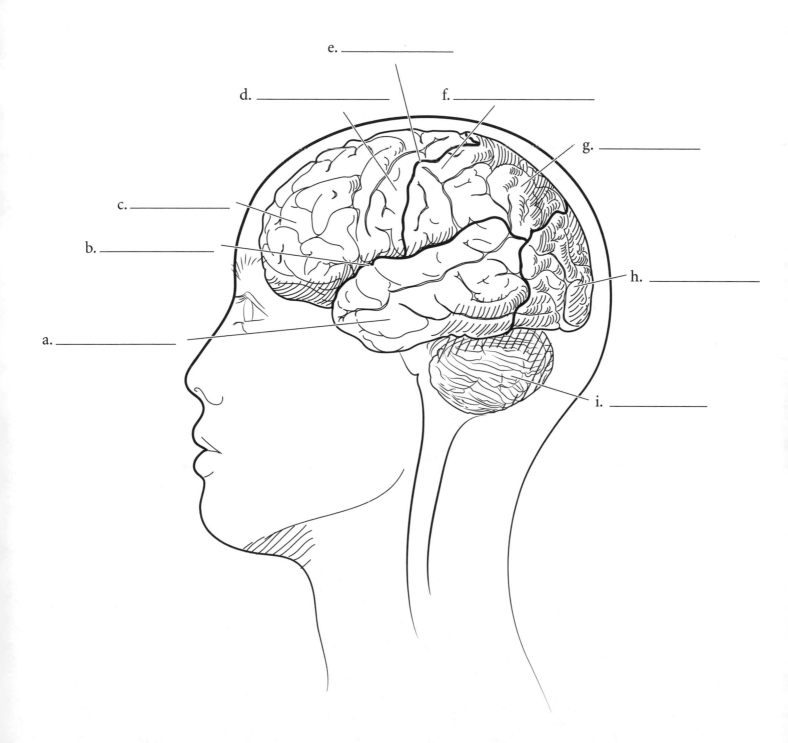

Answer Key: a. Temporal lobe, b. Lateral fissure, c. Frontal lobe, d. Precentral gyrus, e. Central sulcus, f. Postcentral gyrus, g. Parietal lobe, h. Occipital lobe, i. Cerebellum

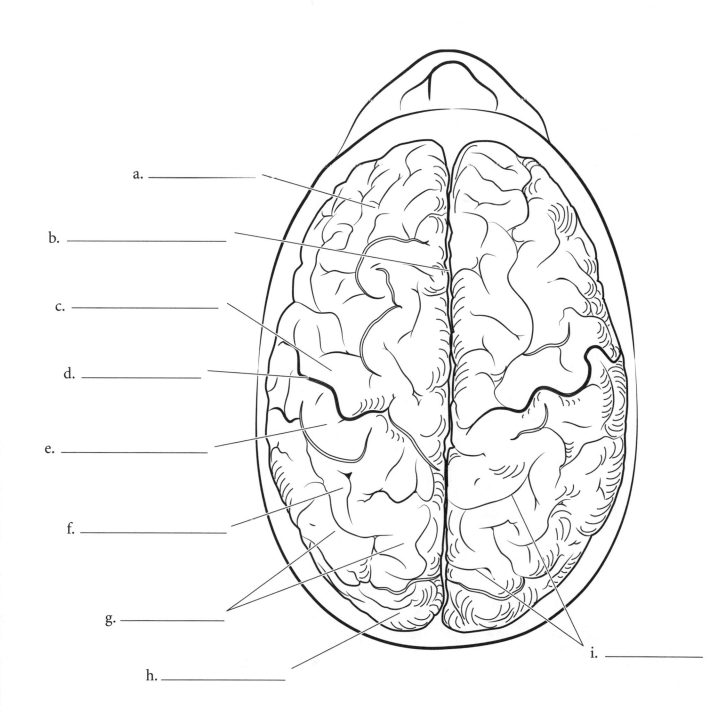

SUPERIOR ASPECT OF THE BRAIN

From the superior aspect, the two **cerebral hemispheres** are divided by the **longitudinal fissure**. The **frontal lobes** are separated from the **parietal lobe** by the **central sulcus**. The **precentral gyrus (primary motor cortex)** and the **postcentral gyrus (primary somatosensory cortex)** are on either side of the central sulcus. The **gyri** are the raised areas of the cerebral cortex and the **sulci** are the shallow depressions of the cerebral cortex. Together, these compose the **convolutions** of the brain. Label and color the regions of the superior aspect of the brain.

a. _____

b. _____

c. _____

d. _____

e. _____

f. _____

g. _____

h. _____

i. _____

Answer Key: a. Frontal lobe, b. Longitudinal fissure, c. Precentral gyrus, d. Central sulcus, e. Postcentral gyrus, f. Parietal lobe, g. Gyri, h. Occipital lobe, i. Sulci

INFERIOR ASPECT OF THE BRAIN

When seen from an inferior view, many different features can be seen on the brain. The **frontal lobe** is anterior and the **temporal lobe** and **cerebellum** are visible as well. The cerebellum has small folds called folia. The **medulla oblongata** is attached to the spinal cord and the **pons** is anterior to the medulla oblongata. Anterior to the pons are the **mammillary bodies** which are responsible for the olfactory (smell) reflex. The **pituitary gland** is next to the mammillary bodies. Anterior to the pituitary is the **optic chiasma**, an x-shaped structure that has the optic nerves anteriorly and the optic tracts posteriorly. The olfactory tracts are seen in this view of the brain as two parallel structures on either side of the longitudinal fissure. The blood vessels of the brain are not visible in this illustration because they obstruct some of the neural structures. They are covered in the cardiovascular section. The cranial nerves will be covered in subsequent pages. Label the structures seen in an inferior view and color them in.

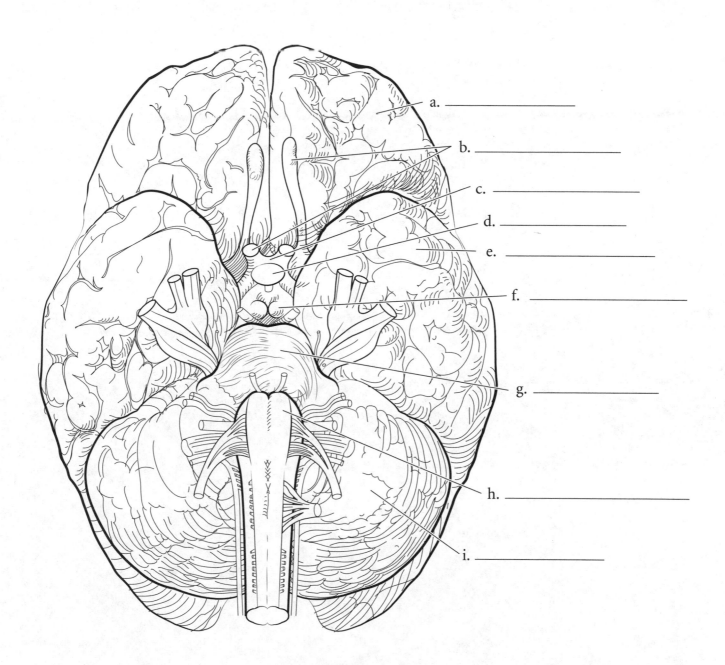

a. _____

b. _____

c. _____

d. _____

e. _____

f. _____

g. _____

h. _____

i. _____

Answer Key: a. Frontal lobe, b. Cranial nerves, c. Optic chiasma, d. Pituitary, e. Temporal lobe, f. Mammillary body, g. Pons, h. Medulla oblongata, i. Cerebellum

MIDSAGITTAL SECTION OF THE BRAIN

When the brain is sectioned in the midsagittal plane, many internal features are visible. One of the most obvious features is the crescent-shaped **corpus callosum**. Superficial to this is the cerebral hemisphere with the **frontal lobe**, **parietal lobe**, and **occipital lobe**. Locate the **thalamus**, **hypothalamus**, and **mammillary body** along with the **optic chiasma** and the **pituitary gland**. The **pineal gland** is a small structure at the posterior aspect of the thalamus. These structures are all part of the forebrain. The midbrain is a small section with the **cerebral peduncles** forming the inferior aspect of the midbrain and the

cerebral **aqueduct** as a narrow tube between the peduncles and the corpora quadrigemina. The corpora consist of the **superior colliculi** which are responsible for visual reflexes and the **inferior colliculi** which are responsible for auditory reflexes. Posterior and inferior to the midbrain is the hindbrain. It consists of the **pons**, the **cerebellum** and the **medulla oblongata**. The pons is a large, oval-shaped structure. The cerebellum is visible with the arbor vitae (white matter of the cerebellum) and a triangular space known as the **fourth ventricle**. The medulla oblongata is the terminal part of the hindbrain. Label the features of the midsagittal section of the brain and color them in.

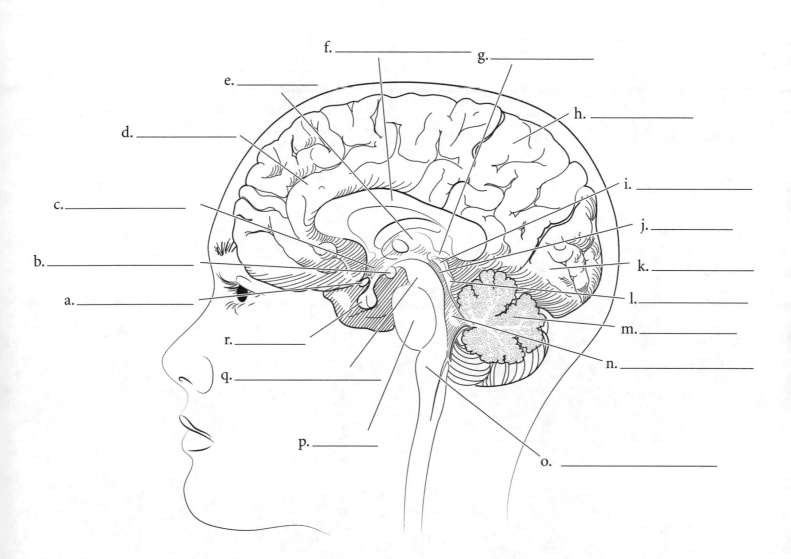

Answer Key: a. Optic chiasma, b. Mammillary body, c. Hypothalamus, d. Frontal lobe, e. Thalamus, f. Corpus callosum, g. Pineal gland, h. Parietal lobe, i. Superior colliculus, j. Cerebral aqueduct, k. Occipital lobe, l. Inferior colliculus, m. Cerebellum, n. Fourth ventricle, o. Medulla oblongata, p. Pons, q. Cerebral peduncle, r. Pituitary

CORONAL SECTION OF THE BRAIN

When the brain is sectioned in the coronal plane, the **convolutions** are obvious. The **gray matter** is on the external aspect of the brain and the **white matter** is internal. There are deep sections of gray matter in the brain and these are known as **basal nuclei**. The external gray matter is known as the **cerebral cortex** and is divided into the **gyri** (raised areas) and **sulci** (depressed areas). The **longitudinal fissure** is the deep cleft that separates the **cerebral hemispheres**. The cerebral hemispheres are connected by the **corpus callosum**. Deep in the hemispheres are spaces known as the **lateral ventricles** and the **third ventricle** is a space in the middle part of the brain. On the sides of the third ventricle is the **thalamus** and the floor of the third ventricle is the hypothalamus. The pituitary is suspended from the hypothalamus by the infundibulum.

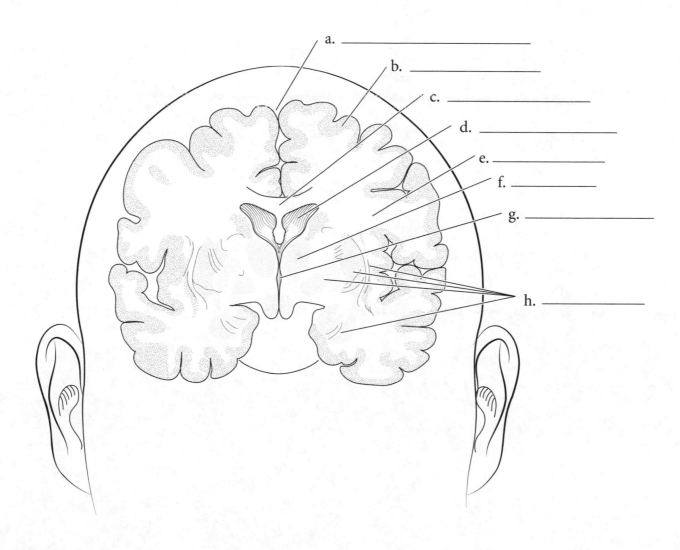

a. _____

b. _____

c. _____

d. _____

e. _____

f. _____

g. _____

h. _____

Answer Key: a. Longitudinal fissure, b. Cerebral cortex (gray matter), c. Corpus callosum, d. Lateral ventricle, e. White matter, f. Thalamus, g. Third ventricle, h. Basal nuclei

LIMBIC SYSTEM

The limbic system is deep in the cerebrum and performs numerous functions. The system has an important role in memory and in emotions (both positive and negative). The sense of smell enters the limbic system and has interpretive centers there. The **cingulate gyrus** is a curved part of the system and coordinates sensory input with emotions. The **hippocampus** and **amygdala** are also parts of the limbic system. The amygdala plays a role in both arousal and aversion and the hippocampus is involved in memory formation. The **hippocampal gyrus** is part of the temporal lobe and takes sensory information to the hippocampus. Memory apparently enters the limbic system as damage to the limbic system impairs memory formation. The storage of memory occurs in other parts of the brain. The **mammillary body** receives olfactory inputs and the **fornix** connects the mammillary body to the hippocampus. Label and color the parts of the limbic system.

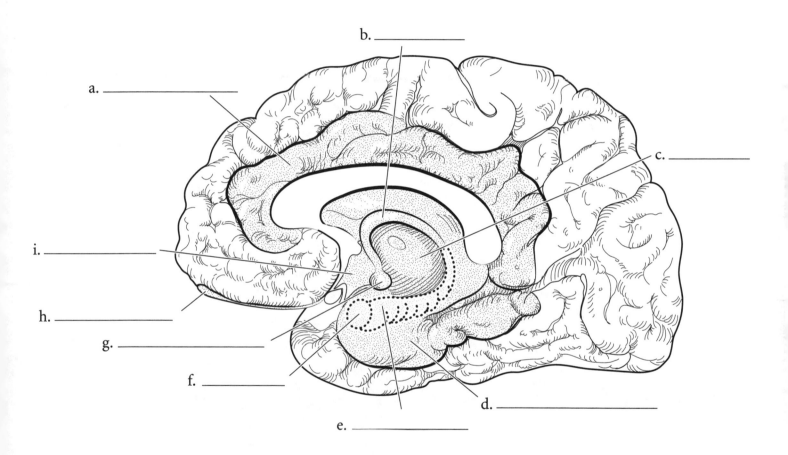

Answer Key: a. Cingulate gyrus, b. Fornix, c. Thalamus, d. Hippocampal gyrus, e. Hippocampus, f. Amygdala, g. Mammillary body, h. Olfactory bulb, i. Hypothalamus

FUNCTIONAL AREAS OF THE CEREBRUM

The cerebrum can be described not only physically but also in terms of the functional areas. The functions of language are many and have different areas of specialization. The **motor speech area** (**Broca's area**) is typically on the left side of the frontal lobe and it involves the formation of words. Coordination of the tongue and other parts of the vocal apparatus occur here. **Wernicke's area** is located in the parieto-temporal region and is involved in the syntax of speech. Wernicke's area allows for the formation of sentence structure while Broca's area is involved in the articulation of speech.

The **primary motor cortex** is located in the **precentral gyrus** and it determines what body muscles to move. The **motor association area** is just anterior to the primary motor cortex. The **primary somatosensory cortex** receives sensory information from the body and has a sensory association area just posterior to it. On the inferior part of the **postcentral gyrus** is the **primary gustatory cortex**. Here is where the sense of taste is interpreted.

The posterior part of the brain includes the **visual association area**. If this area is damaged, then sight can be impaired or lost completely. The **angular gyrus** is one of the areas associated with reading. The temporal lobe includes the **primary auditory cortex** and the **auditory association area**. Label these functional areas of the brain and color each one in a different color. You may want to use different shades of colors for related areas. For example, you may want to color the primary motor cortex with one shade of green and the related motor association area with another shade of green.

a. _____

b. _____

c. _____

d. _____

e. _____

f. _____

g. _____

h. _____

i. _____

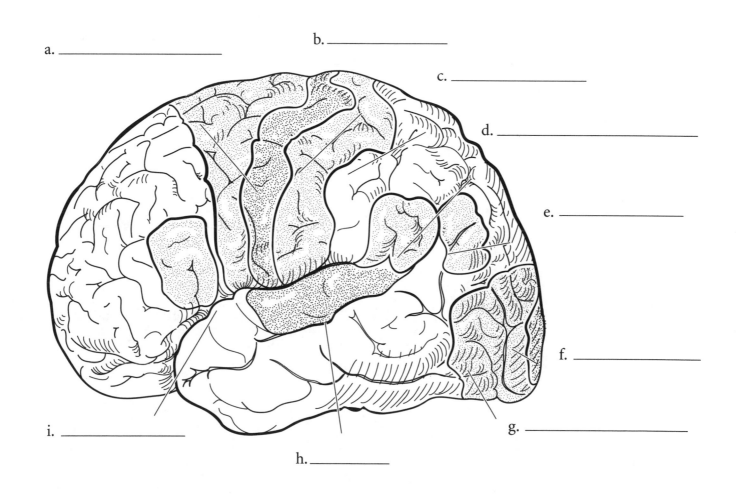

Answer Key: a. Motor association area, b. Primary motor cortex, c. Primary somatosensory cortex, d. Wernicke's area, e. Angular (reading) gyrus, f. Visual area, g. Visual association, h. Auditory cortex, i. Motor speech

VENTRICLES

The brain has hollow cavities enclosed in nervous tissue called ventricles. Each cerebral hemisphere has a **lateral ventricle** and these lead into a central **third ventricle** via the **interventricular foramina**. Cerebrospinal fluid (CSF) is produced from blood capillaries called choroid plexuses in the ventricles and this fluid flows slowly through the ventricles. There are choroid plexuses in all of the ventricles of the brain. The CSF from the lateral ventricles flows into the third ventricle. From the third ventricle the CSF flows into the **cerebral aqueduct** to the **fourth ventricle** which is located anterior to the cerebellum. From the fourth ventricle, CSF exits to the space between the brain and the skull. CSF cushions the brain from mechanical damage and 'floats' the brain in a fluid medium. The CSF is returned to the cardiovascular system by venous sinuses. Label the ventricles, foramina, and the mesencephalic aqueduct. Color in the spaces after you have labeled them.

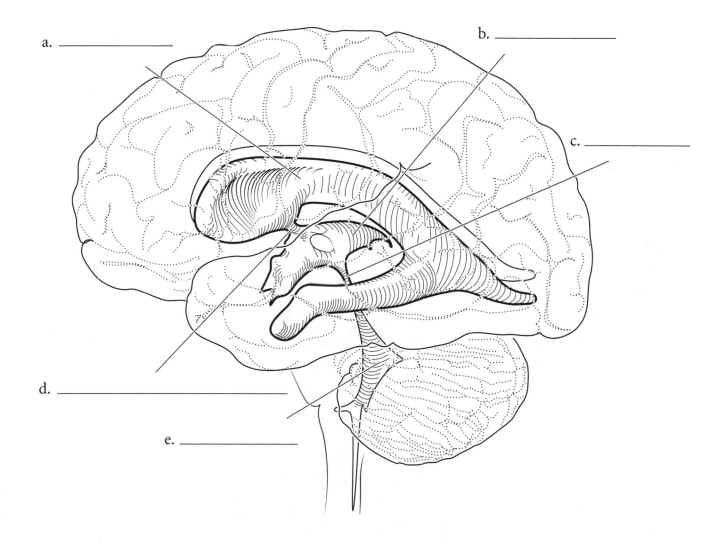

a. _____

b. _____

c. _____

d. _____

e. _____

Answer Key: a. Lateral ventricle, b. Third ventricle, c. Cerebral aqueduct, d. Interventricular foramen, e. Fourth ventricle

CEREBROSPINAL FLUID PATHWAY

Both the brain and spinal cord have layers that cover the nervous tissue. These are known as the meninges. The cerebrospinal fluid (CSF) is produced in the choroid plexuses and then exits to the outside of the brain where it is absorbed in the venous sinus. Label and color the structures and trace the flow of cerebrospinal fluid in the schematic from its source to its reabsorption in the cardiovascular system.

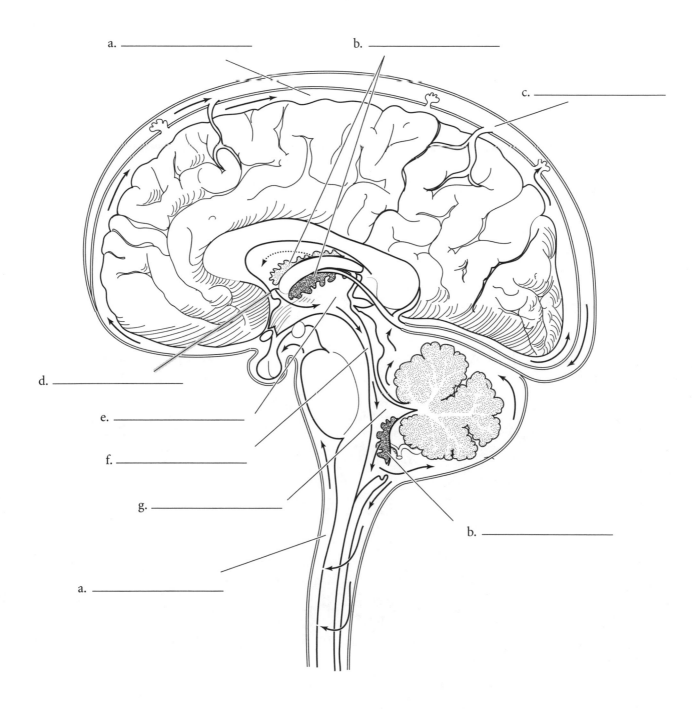

a. _____

b. _____

c. _____

d. _____

e. _____

f. _____

g. _____

b. _____

a. _____

Answer Key: a. Cerebrospinal fluid, b. Choroid plexus, c. Venous sinus, d. Interventricular foramen, e. Third ventricle, f. Cerebral aqueduct, g. Fourth ventricle

SPINAL CORD

The spinal cord is attached to the brain at the foramen magnum. It expands just below this junction as the **cervical enlargement**. This enlargement is due to the increased neural connections with the upper extremities. Another increase in the diameter of the cord is the **lumbar enlargement** and it is due to the neural connections with the lower extremities. The end of the cord is the **conus medullaris** and this is found at the region of the first or second lumbar vertebra. The shortness of the spinal cord occurs because it matures early and the vertebral column continues to grow. The neural fibers continue in the vertebral canal as the **cauda equina**, a structure that resembles a horse's tail. The cord is attached to the coccyx by an extension of the pia mater called the **filum terminale**.

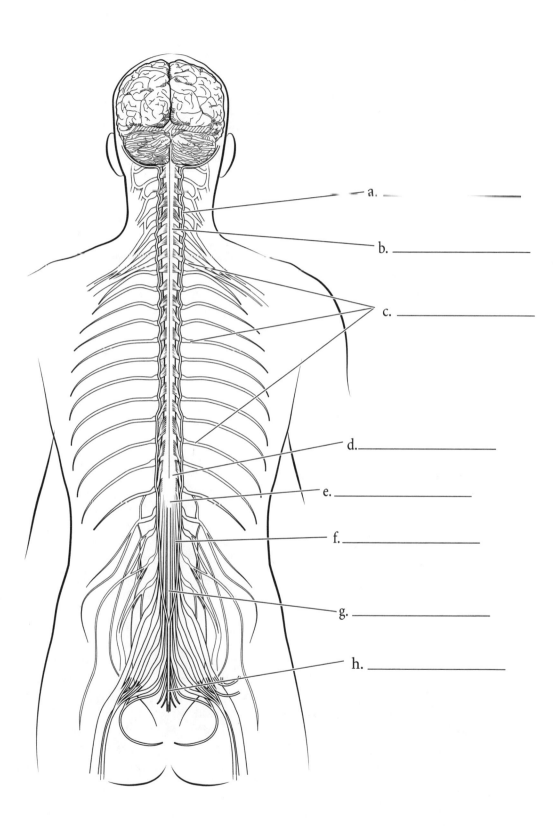

a. _____

b. _____

c. _____

d. _____

e. _____

f. _____

g. _____

h. _____

Answer Key: a. Dura mater, b. Cervical enlargement, c. Spinal nerves, d. Lumbar enlargement, e. Conus medullaris, f. Cauda equina, g. Filum terminale, h. Coccygeal ligament

CRANIAL NERVES

The cranial nerves are those nerves that attach to the brain. They are paired and are numbered (typically by Roman numerals) from anterior to posterior. The **olfactory nerve** is a sensory nerve that receives the sense of smell from the nose and transmits it to the brain. The **optic nerve** takes visual impulses from the eye while the **oculomotor nerve** mostly takes motor impulses to several muscles that move the eye. The **trochlear nerve** takes motor impulses to the superior oblique muscle. The trochlear nerve is so named because it innervates a muscle that passes through a loop called the trochlea. The **trigeminal nerve** is a large nerve located laterally in the pons. It is a mixed nerve (having both sensory and motor functions) that has three branches. The ophthalmic branch innervates the upper head while the maxillary branch innervates the region around the maxilla. The mandibular branch innervates the jaw. The **abducens nerve** is posterior to the trigeminal and is located exiting the brain between the pons and the medulla oblongata. It is a motor nerve to the lateral rectus muscle of the eye. On the anterior portion of the medulla oblongata is the **facial nerve**, which is both a sensory and motor nerve to the face and the tongue. The **vestibulocochlear nerve** is a sensory nerve that receives impulses from the ear. It picks up auditory stimuli as well as information about equilibrium. The **glossopharyngeal nerve** is a nerve that carries both sensory and motor impulses. It innervates the tongue and throat. A large nerve on the side of the medulla oblongata is the **vagus nerve**. It is also a mixed nerve carrying both sensory and motor impulses. The vagus nerve innervates organs in the thoracic and abdominal regions. The **accessory nerve** is inferior to the vagus nerve and is a motor nerve to the neck muscles. The **hypoglossal nerve** is a motor nerve to the tongue. Label the cranial nerves and color each pair a different color.

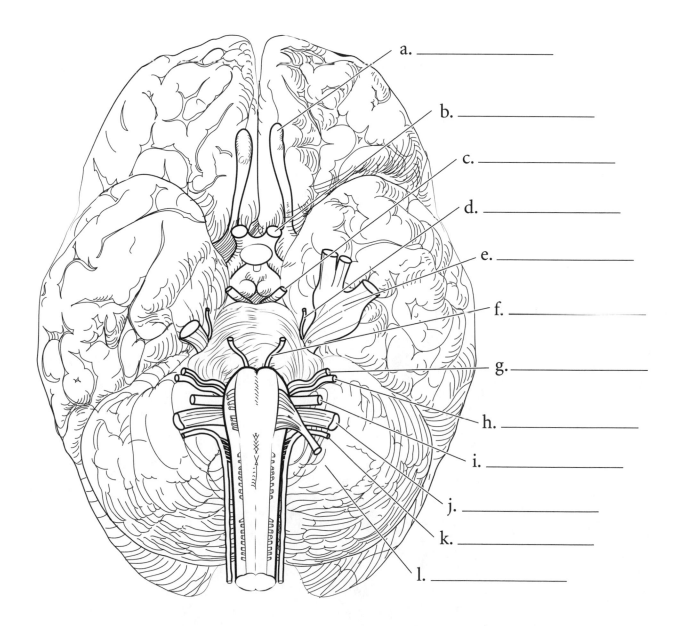

a. _____

b. _____

c. _____

d. _____

e. _____

f. _____

g. _____

h. _____

i. _____

j. _____

k. _____

l. _____

Answer Key: a. Olfactory, b. Optic, c. Oculomotor, d. Trochlear, e. Trigeminal, f. Abducens, g. Facial, h. Vestibulocochlear, i. Glossopharyngeal, j. Vagus, k. Accessory, l. Hypoglossal

SPINAL CORD AND SPINAL NERVES

When seen in cross section, the spinal cord is composed of an internal arrangement of gray matter resembling a butterfly and an external white matter. The two thin strips of gray matter are the **posterior gray horns** and the more rounded sections are the **anterior gray horns**. The **lateral gray horns** are found in the thoracic and lumbar regions. The hole in the middle of the spinal cord is the **central canal** and the gray matter that surrounds the central canal is the gray commissure. The spinal cord has two main depressions in it, the **posterior median sulcus** and the **anterior median fissure**. Label the parts of the spinal cord and color in the regions.

Attached to the spinal cord are the **spinal nerves** that take impulses from the spinal cord to the peripheral nerves and impulses to the spinal cord. The **spinal nerves** are mixed nerves that pass through the intervertebral foramina of the vertebral column. The spinal nerve splits into a **dorsal root** and a **ventral root**. The dorsal root ganglion is a swelling of the dorsal root within its intervertebral foramen. The dorsal root ganglion contains the nerve cell bodies of the sensory neurons coming from the body. The ganglion leads to the **dorsal root** which branches into the **rootlets**. These branches carry sensory information to the **posterior gray horn** of the spinal cord. The ventral root carries motor information from the **anterior gray horn** and innervates muscles.

Both the brain and spinal cord have layers that cover the nervous tissue. These are known as the **meninges** and there are three layers. The outermost layer is the **dura mater** and it is a tough connective tissue layer. Underneath this layer is the **arachnoid mater**, which is so named because it looks like a spider web. At a deeper layer is the subarachnoid space, which is filled with cerebrospinal fluid. The deepest of the layers is the **pia mater** and it is located on the surface of the nervous tissue. Label the meninges and the structures associated with the spinal cord in both the horizontal view and the lateral view and color them in.

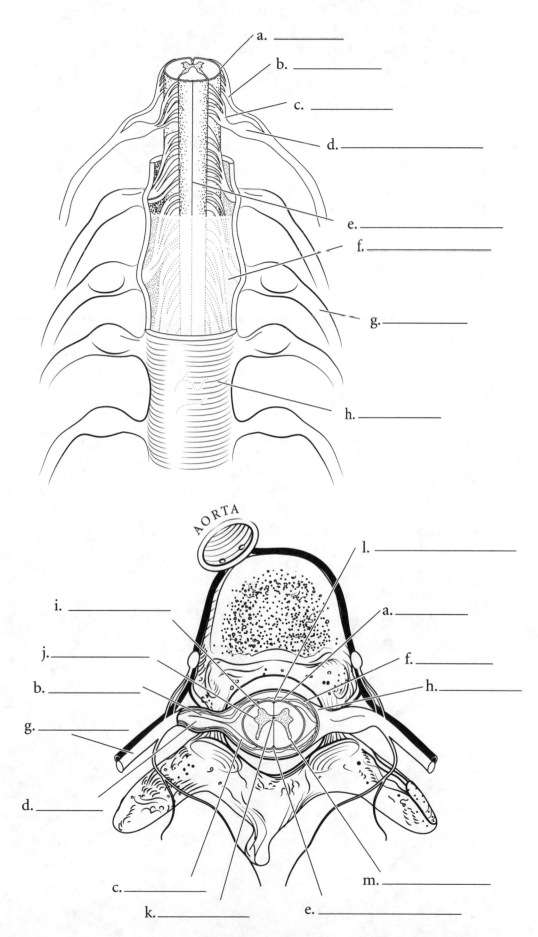

Answer Key: a. Pia mater, b. Ventral root, c. Dorsal root, d. Dorsal root ganglion, e. Posterior median sulcus, f. Arachnoid, g. Spinal nerve, h. Dura mater, i. Anterior gray horn, j. Lateral gray horn, k. Central canal, l. Anterior median fissure, m. Posterior gray horn

PLEXUSES AND THORACIC NERVES

There are 31 pairs of spinal nerves grouped by region of the vertebral column. The **cervical nerves** are the most superior and there are eight pairs of them. The first cervical nerves arise superior to the first cervical vertebra. The **thoracic nerves** arise as twelve pairs. They lead to nerves that innervate the muscles between the ribs and associated skin. There are five pairs of **lumbar nerves** and five pairs of **sacral nerves**. The last pair of spinal nerves is the **coccygeal nerves**.

A **plexus** is a web-like arrangement of nerves that is near the spinal cord and gives rise to the **terminal nerves**. The most superior plexus is the

cervical plexus which arises from the first five cervical spinal nerves. The **brachial plexus** receives input from the fifth through eighth cervical nerves and the first pair of thoracic nerves. The **lumbar plexus** arises from the first four pairs of lumbar nerves and the **sacral plexus** is associated with the last two pairs of lumbar nerves and the first four pairs of sacral nerves. Sometimes the lumbar and sacral plexuses are grouped together as the **lumbosacral plexus**. Use one color to color in the short segments of the spinal nerves and label the plexuses. Color each plexus a different color.

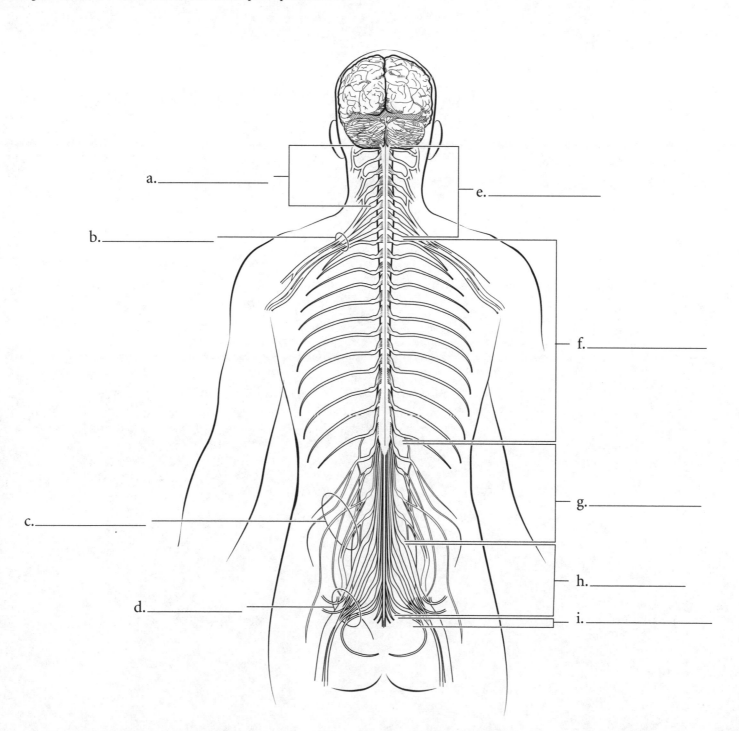

Answer Key: a. Cervical plexus, b. Brachial plexus, c. Lumbar plexus, d. Sacral plexus, e. Cervical nerves, f. Thoracic nerves, g. Lumbar nerves, h. Sacral nerves, i. Coccygeal nerves

NERVES OF CERVICAL PLEXUS

The **cervical plexus** is a complex interweaving of branches from the first five pairs of cervical nerves. The **hypoglossal nerve** enters this plexus from the head. The **ansa cervicalis** is an arched structure (*ansa* is Latin for loop) that has many nerves innervating the anterior throat muscles. The major nerves of the cervical plexus are the two **phrenic nerves** that descend to the diaphragm and stimulate the diaphragm to contract. Label the major features of the cervical plexus and color the hypoglossal nerve, the ansa cervicalis, and the phrenic nerve.

Contributions to the accessory nerve leave the cervical plexus from C2, 3, and 4.

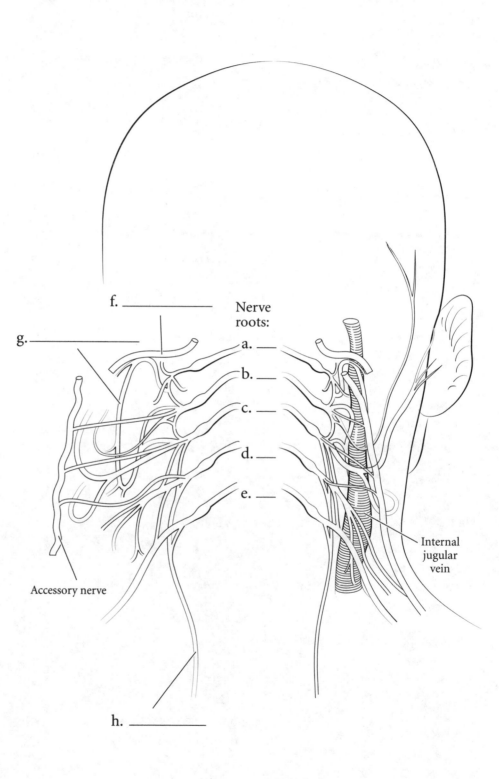

f. _____

Nerve roots:

g. _____

a. ___

b. ___

c. ___

d. ___

e. ___

Internal jugular vein

Accessory nerve

h. _____

NERVES OF BRACHIAL PLEXUS

The brachial plexus is associated with spinal nerves C4–8 and T1. It leads to major nerves of the shoulder and arm. The **axillary nerve** arises from the brachial plexus and innervates the deltoid and the teres minor muscles. It also receives stimulation from the skin of the shoulder and lateral upper limb. The **radial nerve** innervates the triceps brachii muscle and the extensors of the forearm and hand. The **musculocutaneous nerve** innervates the anterior muscles of the arm (biceps brachii, brachialis, and coracobrachialis) and the skin on the lateral side of the forearm. The median nerve runs the length of the arm and forearm and innervates the anterior muscles of the forearm and the muscles associated with the thumb. The **ulnar nerve** passes along the posterior side of the medial epicondyle of the humerus and gives that tingling sensation of the "funny bone" when hit. It innervates the muscles of the medial side of the anterior hand. Label these nerves and related structures and color them in. Select a different color for each nerve.

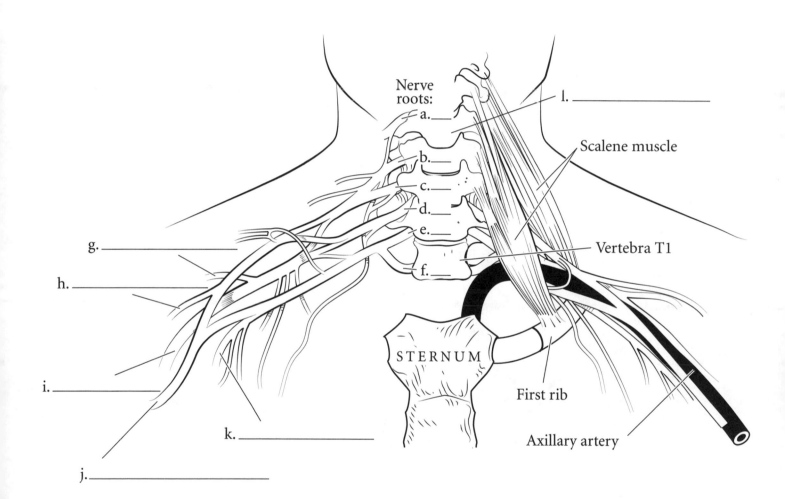

Answer Key: a. C4, b. C5, c. C6, d. C7, e. C8, f. T1, g. Axillary nerve, h. Musculocutaneous nerve, i. Radial nerve, j. Median nerve, k. Ulnar nerve, l. Vertebra C4

NERVES OF LUMBAR PLEXUS

The lumbar plexus leads to nerves on the anterior and the medial aspect of the thigh. A large **femoral nerve** arises from the lumbar plexus and innervates the four muscles of the quadriceps femoris group on the anterior thigh. The **obturator nerve** innervates the adductor muscles of the medial thigh and the **genitofemoral nerve** is a sensory nerve that receives impulses from the male scrotal sac and the labia majora in females. The **iliohypogastric nerve** innervates the muscles of the abdomen and the skin of the belly. The **ilioinguinal nerve** innervates the same muscles as does the iliohypogastric nerve and it receives sensory information from the base of the penis and the scrotum in males, and from the labia majora in females. The **lateral femoral cutaneous nerve** receives sensory information from the skin of the lateral thigh. Label these nerves in the illustration and color them in with a different color.

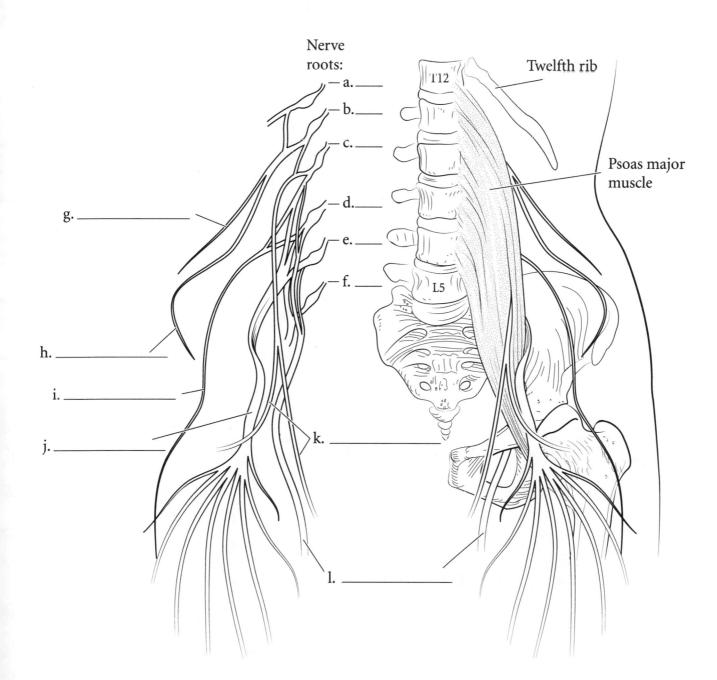

NERVES OF SACRAL PLEXUS

The sacral plexus has nerves that provide genital innervation and also has motor nerves to the posterior hip, thigh, and anterior and posterior leg. The **pudendal nerve** innervates the penis and scrotum in males, the clitoris, labia, and distal vagina in females, and the muscles of the pelvic floor in both sexes. The sacral plexus also has the **superior** and **inferior gluteal nerves** that innervate the gluteal muscles and the **tibial nerve** and the **common fibular nerve**. These last two nerves are grouped together as the **sciatic nerve**, a large nerve of the posterior thigh. The tibial nerve innervates the hamstring muscles, the muscles of the calf, and the muscles originating on the foot. The common fibular nerve innervates the short head of the biceps femoris muscle, the muscles on the lateral side of the leg and the anterior surface of the leg. **Cutaneous branches** innervate the skin and **muscular branches** take motor information to the muscles. Label these nerves and color them in.

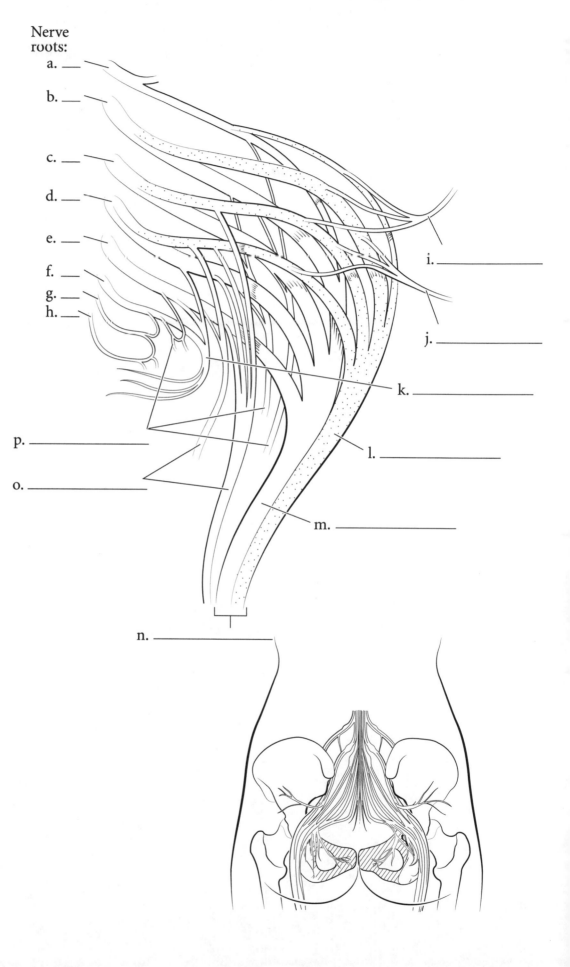

Nerve roots:

a. ____
b. ____
c. ____
d. ____
e. ____
f. ____
g. ____
h. ____

i. ____
j. ____
k. ____
l. ____
m. ____
n. ____
o. ____
p. ____

Answer Key: a. L4, b. L5, c. S1, d. S2, e. S3, f. S4, g. S5, h. Coccygeal nerve, i. Superior gluteal nerve, j. Inferior gluteal nerve, k. Pudendal nerve, l. Common fibular nerve, m. Tibial nerve, n. Sciatic nerve, o. Cutaneous branches, p. Muscular branches

DERMATOMES

Dermatomes are regions of the skin innervated by nerves. The nerves receive sensory inputs from the skin and take that information back to the spinal cord. The clinical importance of dermatomes is the role they play in assessing spinal cord damage. If there is a significant spinal cord injury, then the regions below the level of the injury may not transmit sensory signals to the brain. Lack of sensation in specific areas of the skin provides a base of understanding of where the trauma may be located. Color in the regions that are innervated by the cervical nerves with one color and choose separate colors for the thoracic, lumbar, and sacral innervation. Label the innervations of the dermatomes.

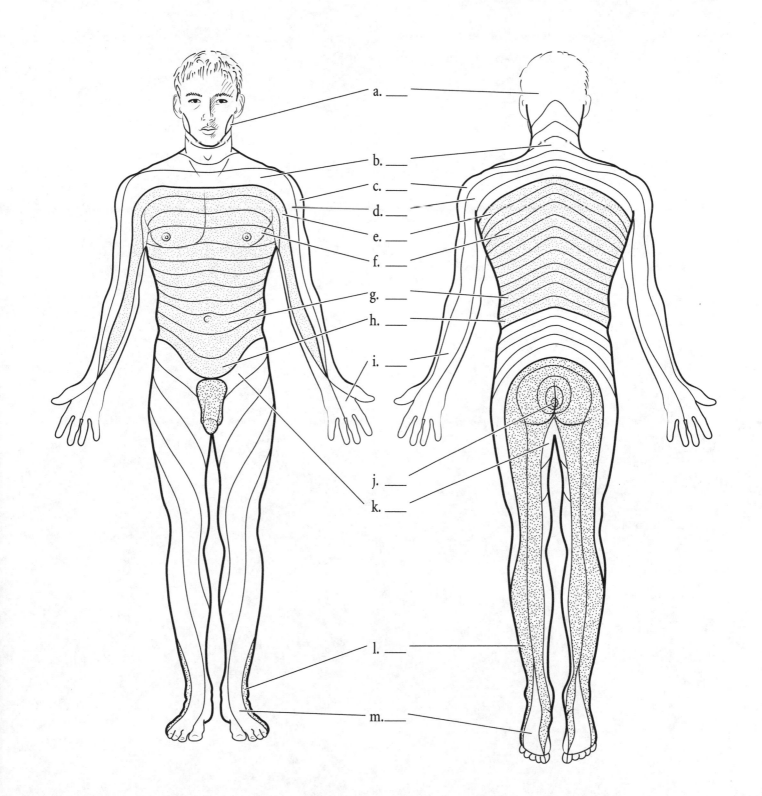

a. ____
b. ____
c. ____
d. ____
e. ____
f. ____
g. ____
h. ____
i. ____
j. ____
k. ____
l. ____
m. ____

Answer Key: a. C2, b. C5, c. C6, d. C7, e. T1, f. T4, g. T10, h. T12, i. C7, j. S5, k. L1, l. S1, m. L5

AUTONOMIC NERVOUS SYSTEM—SYMPATHETIC DIVISION

The **autonomic nervous system (ANS)** regulates automatic functions of the human body. Changes in heart rate, pupil dilation, digestive functions, and blood flow to the kidney are all controlled by the ANS. There is some possibility of conscious regulation of parts of the ANS, but, for the most part, it functions without conscious control. There are two divisions of the autonomic nervous system. The resting state of the body is controlled by the **parasympathetic division**. Digestion, kidney filtration, erection of the clitoris, erection of the penis, and pupil constriction are some of the functions of the parasympathetic division. This division is also known as the **craniosacral division** because the nerves exit the central nervous system (CNS) in these locations. The cranial segments go to the eye, salivary glands, heart, lung, digestive system, and kidneys. The sacral segments go to the lower digestive tract, bladder, and reproductive organs.

The **sympathetic division** controls the "fight or flight" response of the body, shutting down the digestive functions, inhibiting erections, shunting blood away from the kidneys, and dilating the pupils. The sympathetic division increases heart rate, dilates capillaries in the lungs, brain and muscle tissue, and stimulates the adrenal glands. This division is also known as the **thoracolumbar division** because the nerves exit the CNS in the thoracic and lumbar regions of the spinal cord. There are ganglia associated with the sympathetic division and these are located on either side of the ventral portion of the vertebral column. They are called the **sympathetic chain ganglia** and the neurons from the thoracolumbar division synapse with nerve cells in these ganglia.

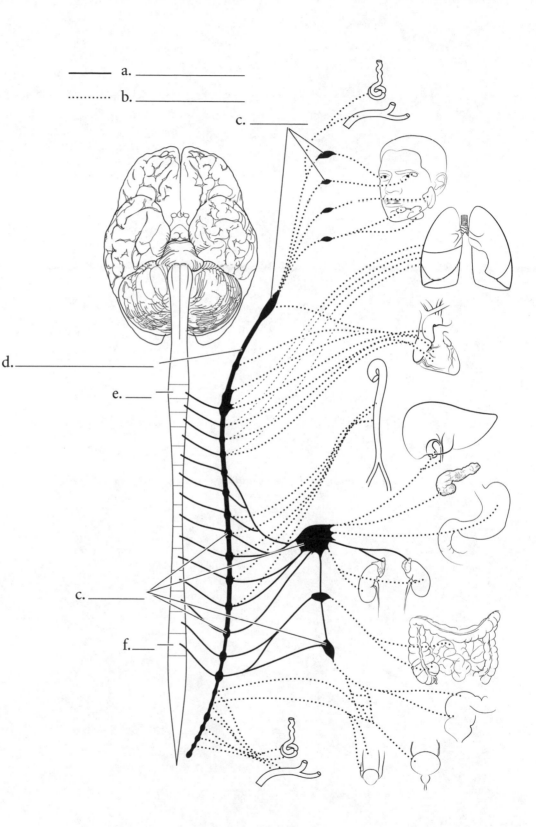

a. _____
b. _____
c. _____
d. _____
e. _____
c. _____
f. _____

Answer Key: a. Preganglionic, b. Postganglionic, c. Ganglia, d. Sympathetic trunk, e. T1, f. L2

AUTONOMIC NERVOUS SYSTEM— PARASYMPATHETIC DIVISION

The parasympathetic and sympathetic divisions are antagonistic to one another and organs under the influence of the ANS have dual innervation. Typically, one division either inhibits the organ from functioning or causes an increase in activity in the organ. This occurs due to the difference in neurotransmitters secreted by the separate divisions. At the terminal end of the para-sympathetic division, the neurotransmitter is acetylcholine. At the terminal end of the sympathetic division, the neurotransmitter is mostly norepinephrine.

The neurons leaving the CNS are called **preganglionic neurons**. In the case of the parasympathetic division, the preganglionic neurons secrete acetylcholine as neurotransmitters. The **ganglia** of the parasympathetic division are next to, or in, the organ they innervate. The **postganglionic neurons** secrete acetylcholine as well. In the sympathetic division, the preganglionic neurons secrete acetylcholine in the sympathetic chain ganglia. The postganglionic neurons mostly secrete norepinephrine to stimulate or inhibit the organs they innervate.

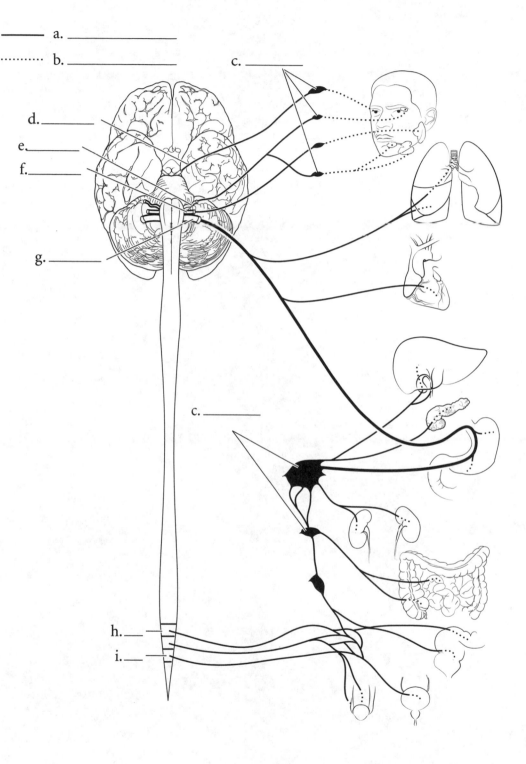

a. _____
b. _____
c. _____
d. _____
e. _____
f. _____
g. _____
c. _____
h. _____
i. _____

Answer Key: a. Preganglionic, b. Postganglionic, c. Ganglia, d. Oculomotor III, e. Facial VII, f. Glossopharyngeal IX, g. Vagus X, h. S2, i. S4

SKIN RECEPTORS

There are several sense receptors in the skin. Some of these are involved in determining mechanical vibration, some sense temperature, and some sense pain. The receptors for mechanical vibration pick up light touch or are involved in perception of pressure. There are **hair receptors** that wrap around the hair follicles, and as the hair moves it stimulates the neurons. Light touch is perceived by both **Meissner's corpuscles** and

Merkel's disks. These receptors are found in the superficial layers of the skin (**epidermis** and upper **dermis**). In the deeper layers are the **Pacinian** or **lamellated corpuscles** that pick up pressure. **Pain receptors** are located throughout the skin and pick up variable stimuli including extreme temperatures, acids, strong mechanical vibration, etc. Other receptors in the skin are thermoreceptors that pick up the sensation of smaller changes in temperature. Label these structures and color them on the figure.

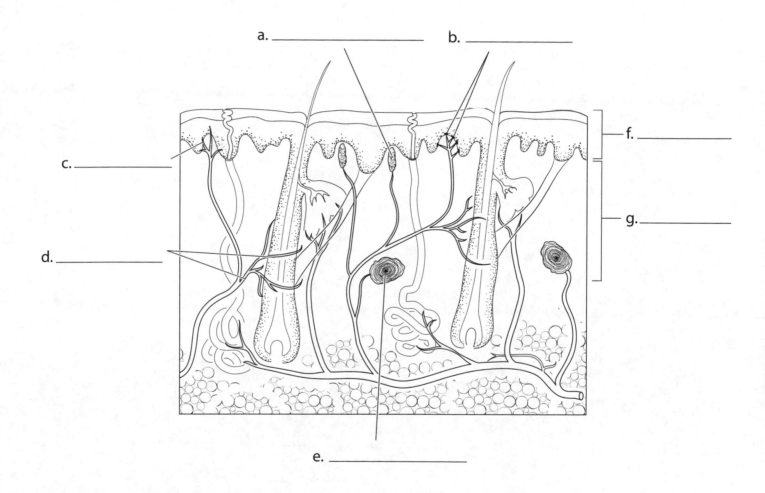

Answer Key: a. Meissner's corpuscles, b. Merkel's disks, c. Pain receptor, d. Hair receptors, e. Pacinian (lamellated) corpuscle, f. Epidermis, g. Dermis

TONGUE

The tongue is the region where taste is perceived. The tongue has regions that are sensitive to different tastes and these vary from person to person. Not only do people taste material in different places on the tongue, but the sensitivity to taste is different in individuals. Taste buds are located on the sides of papillae of the tongue. The **lingual tonsils** are found on the posterior tongue and the **palatine tonsils** are on the sides of the oral cavity. Posterior and inferior to the tongue is the **epiglottis**. The papillae of the tongue come in a few shapes. **Vallate papillae** are shaped like mesas. They have a flat top. **Filiform papillae** are line-shaped while **fungiform papillae** are shaped like mushrooms. Label and color the papillae.

a. _____

b. _____

c. _____

d. _____

e. _____

f. _____

Color in the **taste buds** in the illustration. They consist of epithelial cells and nerve cells. Taste is sensed if the material to be tasted is in solution and comes into contact with the **taste pore**. The taste buds have taste hairs that extend into the taste pore and connect with taste cells that in turn synapse with **sensory nerve fibers** that take the sense of taste to the brain. Label the figure and color in the various structures.

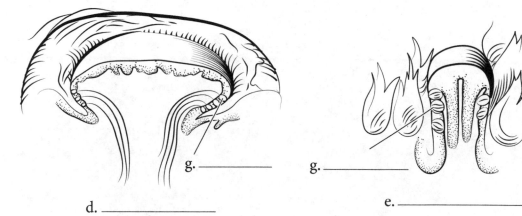

g. _____

d. _____

g. _____

e. _____

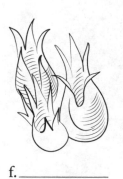

f. _____

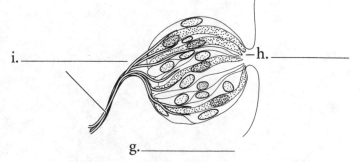

i. _____

h. _____

g. _____

Answer Key: a. Epiglottis, b. Palatine tonsil, c. Lingual tonsil, d. Vallate papilla, e. Fungiform papilla, f. Filiform papillae, g. Taste bud, h. Taste pore, i. Sensory nerve fibers

NOSE

The sense of smell is more complex than the sense of taste. There are only five primary tastes but many different kinds of smells. The region that is sensitive to smell is the **olfactory epithelium** which is located in the superior portion of the **nasal cavity**. The olfactory epithelium consists of elongated epithelial cells that are **supporting cells** with neurons called **olfactory cells**. These olfactory cells have **olfactory hairs** on their surface. Chemicals that are inhaled come into contact with a mucous sheet and are picked up by the olfactory cells. The sensation of smell is transmitted by the olfactory nerves through the **cribriform plate** of the ethmoid bone and they synapse in the **olfactory bulb** at the base of the frontal lobe of the brain.

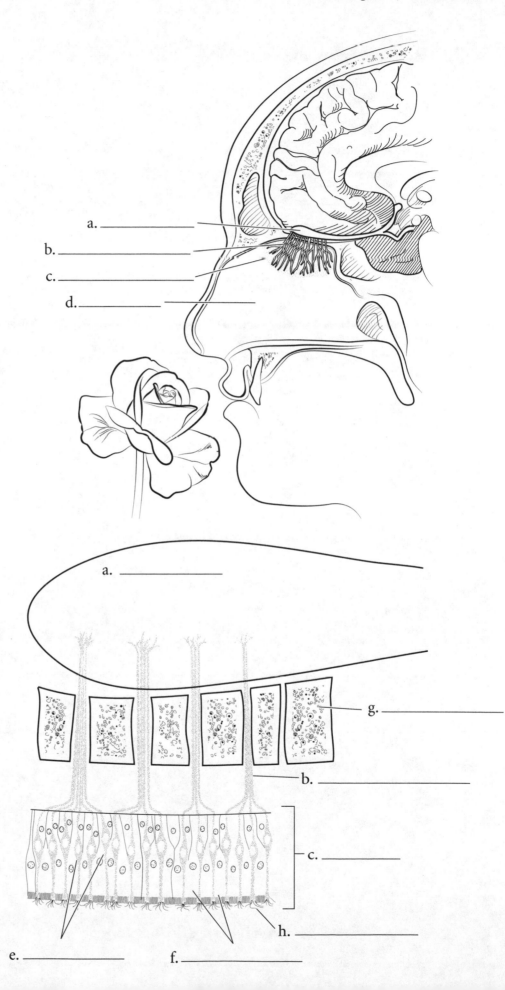

a. _____
b. _____
c. _____
d. _____

a. _____
g. _____
b. _____
c. _____
h. _____
e. _____
f. _____

Answer Key: a. Olfactory bulb,
b. Olfactory filaments,
c. Olfactory epithelium
d. Nasal cavity, e. Olfactory cells,
f. Supporting cells, g. Cribriform plate,
h. Olfactory hairs

ANTERIOR SURFACE OF THE EYE AND LACRIMAL APPARATUS

The eye is located in the orbit of the skull and has several external features. Above the eye is the **eyebrow**. The corners of the eye have either a **lateral commissure** or a **medial commissure**. Next to the medial commissure is the **caruncle**, a small thickened tissue in the medial corner of the eye. The outer surface of the eye is protected by the **upper** and **lower eyelids.** The blink reflex rapidly closes the eyelids to keep dust from hitting the outer surface of the eye. Label and color the **sclera** (the white of the eye), **iris** (the colored part of the eye), **pupil** (the opening that lets light into the back of the eye), and the eyelids. There is a transparent extension of the sclera called the cornea and it covers the iris and pupil.

The eyes are kept moist and are subject to potential bacterial infection. Tears have antimicrobial properties and are formed by the **lacrimal gland.** They contain digestive enzymes and wash microbes from the surface of the eye. Tears drain from the eye into the **lacrimal canals.** These canals lead into the **nasolacrimal duct** and then into the **nasal cavity.**

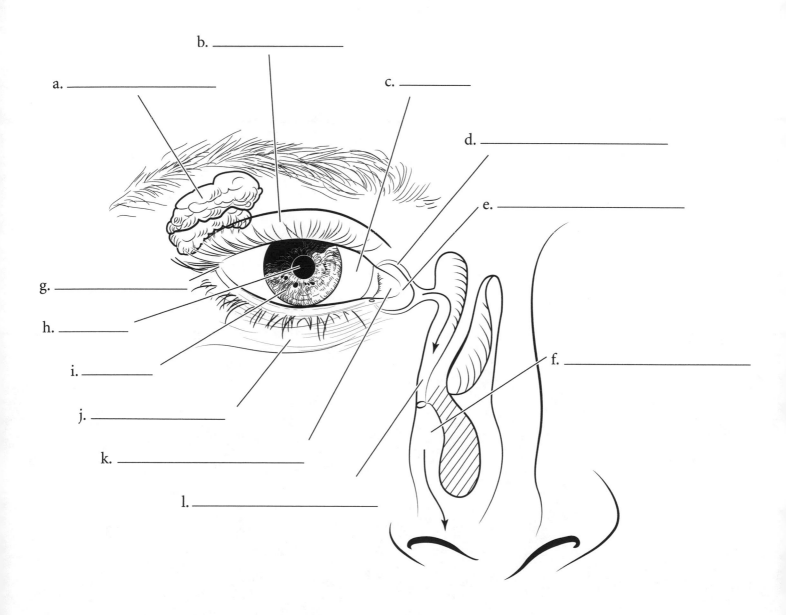

b. _____
a. _____
c. _____
d. _____
e. _____
g. _____
h. _____
i. _____
f. _____
j. _____
k. _____
l. _____

MUSCLES OF THE EYE

The lateral and superior views of the eye show the major muscles controlling the eye. The **lateral rectus** is the muscle that lets you see towards the side. The **medial rectus** turns the eye toward the midline. The **superior rectus** makes you look up while the **inferior rectus** makes you look down. The **superior oblique** turns the eye inferiorly and laterally while the **inferior oblique** makes the eye turn superiorly and laterally. The **levator palpebrae superioris** elevates the eyelid. Label and color the muscles of the eye and the **optic nerve** where it exits the tendinous ring.

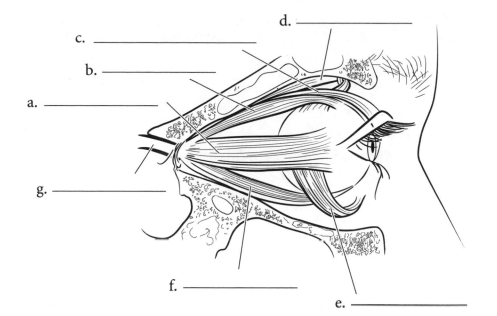

c. _____
d. _____
b. _____
a. _____
g. _____
f. _____
e. _____

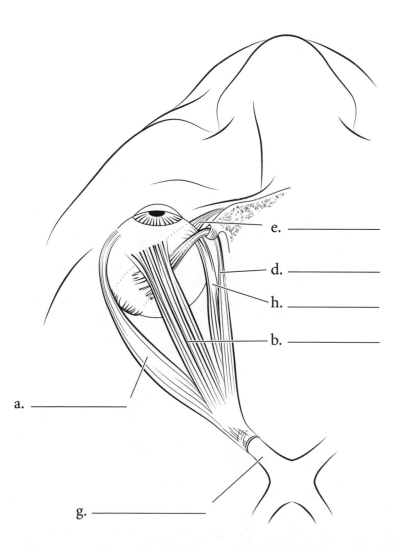

e. _____
d. _____
h. _____
b. _____
a. _____
g. _____

Answer Key: a. Lateral rectus,
b. Superior rectus, c. Levator palpebrae superioris, d. Superior oblique,
e. Inferior oblique, f. Inferior rectus,
g. Optic nerve, h. Medial rectus

MEDIAN SECTION OF THE EYE

The **cornea** is the outermost part of the eye and it is responsible for most of the light refraction in the eye (the bending of light rays). On the periphery of the cornea is the **sclera** which helps maintain eye shape. The space behind the cornea is the **anterior cavity** which is found in front of the **lens**. It is composed of two smaller chambers, the **anterior chamber** and the **posterior chamber**. The anterior chamber is between the cornea and the **iris**, the part that determines eye color. The posterior chamber is between the iris and the **lens**. The lens is made of protein and is held to the wall of the eye by the **suspensory ligaments**. These ligaments are pulled by the **ciliary muscle** on the wall of the eye. When the ligaments tighten, the lens flattens and the eye focuses on distant objects. The fluid in the anterior cavity is known as aqueous humor and it is released by the ciliary body and reabsorbed in the **scleral venous sinus**.

Behind the lens is the **posterior cavity**. This cavity is filled with a jelly-like material called **vitreous humor**. Light travels through this medium to the back of the eye where it strikes the **retina**. The retina is the region of the eye where light waves are converted to nerve impulses. The **fovea** is a small area of the retina where there is a high concentration of cones (cells that determine color and visual acuity.) Behind the retina is the **choroid**, a darkened layer that absorbs light, making vision sharp during the daytime. Behind this layer is the sclera, the white of the eye, where muscles attach. At the posterior of the eye you can see the **optic disk**. This is where the **optic nerve** takes visual impulses from the eye to the brain. Color the median section of the eye after you have filled in the appropriate labels.

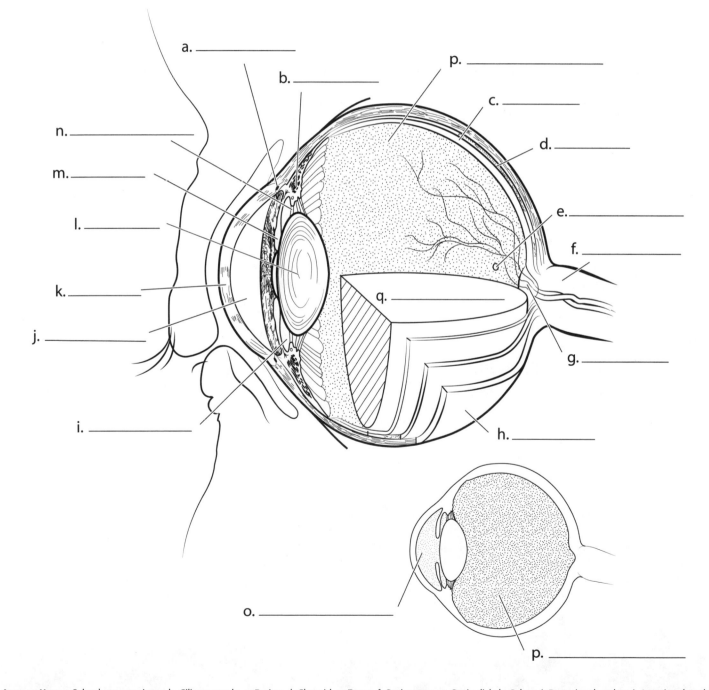

Answer Key: a. Scleral venous sinus , b. Ciliary muscle, c. Retina, d. Choroid, e. Fovea, f. Optic nerve, g. Optic disk, h. Sclera, i. Posterior chamber, j. Anterior chamber, k. Cornea, l. Lens, m. Iris, n. Suspensory ligament, o. Anterior cavity, p. Posterior cavity, q. Vitreous humor

POSTERIOR VIEW OF THE EYE

In the posterior view of the eye you can see the **blood vessels** in the choroid that bring nutrients to the back of the eye. Color these vessels. They enter the eye at a region known as the **optic disk**, which is the same place where the **optic nerve** exits the eye. This is the blind spot of the eye. You should also label and color the **fovea centralis** of the eye and the **macula lutea**. The macula lutea means "yellow body" while the fovea centralis is the region of the eye with a great number of photosensitive cells.

Retina

The retina is the tunic or layer of the eye that converts light energy into nerve impulses. There are two main types of photosensitive cells in the retina. **Rods** are more numerous and they determine motion and night vision. There are many rods in the eye but they are not very sensitive in determining visual detail. This is because many rods connect to one neuron fiber. The other photosensitive cells are **cones**. There are fewer cones per neuron so they produce a sharper visual image. There are three types of cones that have sensitivities to different wavelengths of light. Label and color the rods and cones in the retina.

The retina consists of three layers. The **photoreceptor layer** contains the rods and cones. This is at the posterior layer of the retina. In front of this is the **bipolar layer** that has neurons that synapse with the rods and cones. The layer closest to the posterior cavity is the **ganglionic layer**. The axons of the ganglion cells conduct impulses from the ganglionic layer along the span of the eye and form the **optic nerve**. Label these layers and color them in.

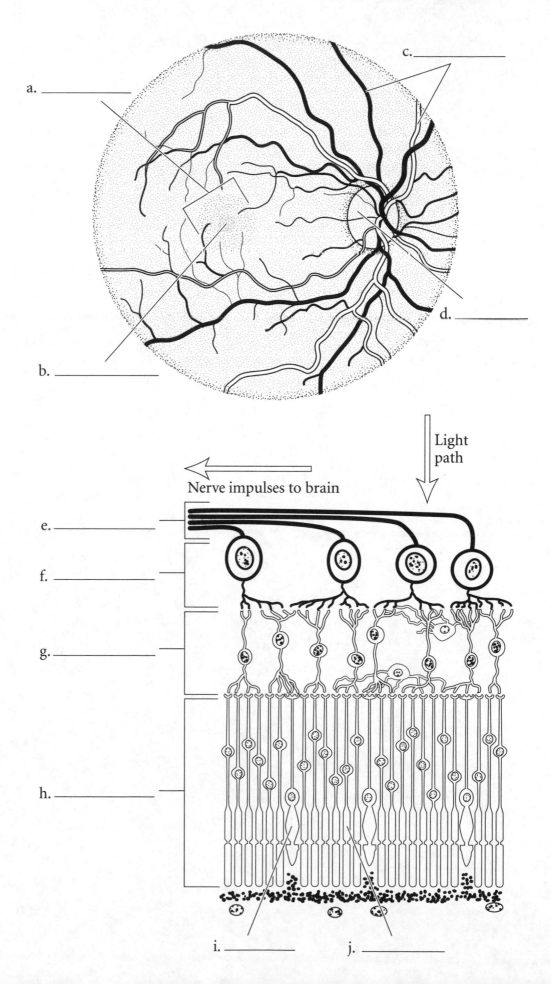

Answer Key: a. Macula lutea, b. Fovea centralis, c. Blood vessels, d. Optic disk e. Optic nerve, f. Ganglionic layer, g. Bipolar layer, h. Photoreceptor layer, i. Cone, j. Rod

OVERVIEW OF EAR

The ear consists of three major regions, the **outer ear**, the **middle ear** and the **inner ear**. The outer ear consists mainly of two parts, the **auricle** (**pinna**), including the **ear lobe** and the **external auditory canal**. The middle ear begins at the **tympanic membrane** (ear drum). Inside the tympanic membrane is the tympanic cavity, another part of the middle ear. Here you should label the ear **ossicles** and the **auditory tube** (Eustachian tube). The inner ear consists of three major regions, the cochlea, the vestibule, and the semicircular ducts. Use a different color for each major region of the ear.

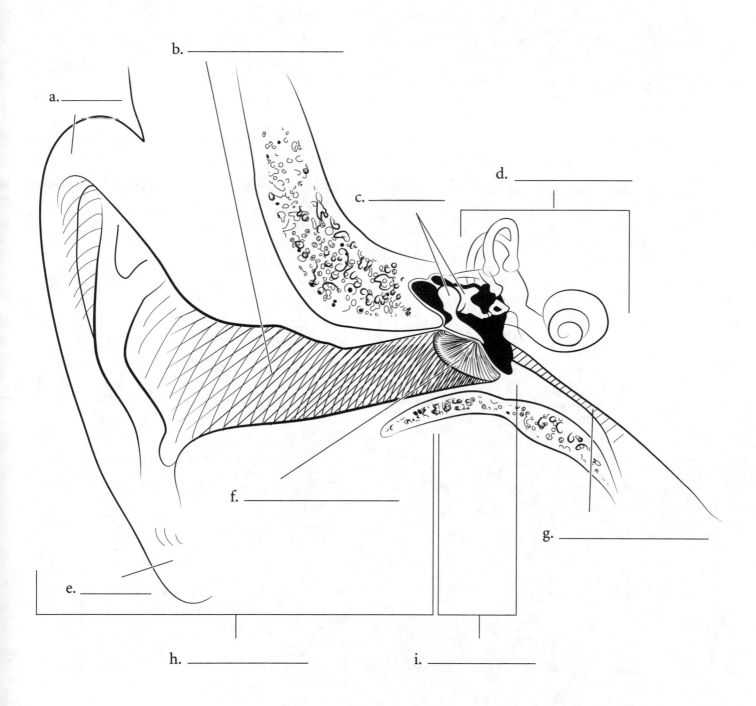

b. _____

a. _____

d. _____

c. _____

f. _____

e. _____

g. _____

h. _____

i. _____

Answer Key: a. Auricle (pinna), b. External auditory canal, c. Ossicles, d. Inner ear, e. Ear lobe, f. Tympanic membrane, g. Auditory tube, h. External ear, i. Middle ear

MIDDLE EAR

The middle ear consists of the **tympanic cavity** and structures in that cavity. It is connected to the nasopharynx by the **auditory tube**. This tube allows for equalization of pressure from the middle ear and the external environment. The three ear ossicles transfer sound from the tympanic membrane to the **oval window** of the inner ear. Label the three ear ossicles, the **malleus, incus,** and **stapes**, and color each one a different color. Color the oval window where the stapes connects and use lighter colors for the auditory tube and the tympanic cavity.

INNER EAR

The inner ear consists of the **cochlea**, the **vestibule**, and the **semicircular ducts**. In Latin, the name *cochlea* means snail shell and it spirals like a snail. Its function is to translate the mechanical vibrations of sound into nerve impulses. The cochlea has an **oval window** that attaches to the stapes and a **round window** that allows for changes in pressure to occur in the inner ear. Label the cochlea and color it in. The vestibule has two parts, the **utricle** and the **saccule**. These are involved in equilibrium. They determine static equilibrium whereby a person can determine the position of the body at rest. They also register acceleration. Color each of these parts of the vestibule a different color. The semicircular ducts respond to angular acceleration. There are three semicircular ducts, the **posterior**, the **anterior**, and the **lateral semicircular ducts**. Color each of the semicircular ducts a different color.

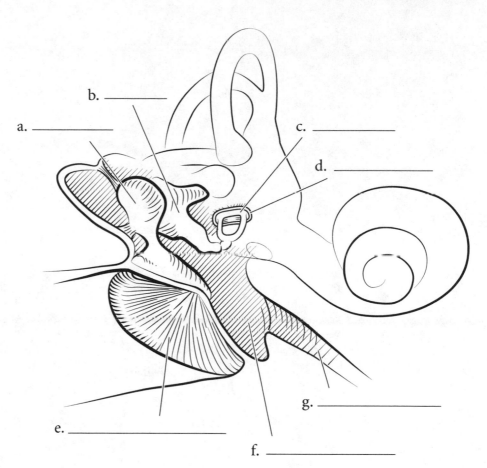

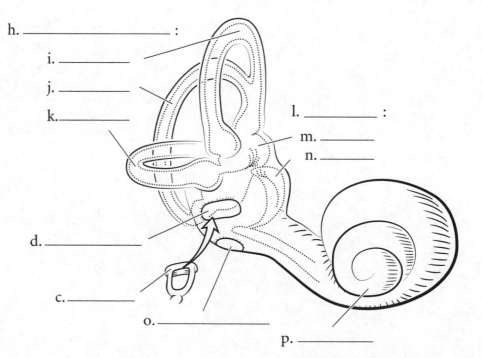

Answer Key: a. Malleus, b. Incus, c. Stapes, d. Oval window, e. Tympanic membrane, f. Tympanic cavity, g. Auditory (Eustachian) tube, h. Semicircular ducts, i. Anterior duct, j. Posterior duct, k. Lateral duct, l. Vestibule, m. Utricle, n. Saccule, o. Round window, p. Cochlea

LABYRINTHS OF THE INNER EAR

The outer part of the inner ear consists of the **bony labyrinth**, an outer encasement of bone. Inside of this is a fluid called **perilymph**. Inside of this is the **membranous labyrinth**. It is filled with a fluid called **endolymph**. Label these structures and fluids.

a. _____ :
b. _____
c. _____
d. _____
e. _____
f. _____
g. _____
h. _____ :
i. _____
j. _____
k. _____
l. _____

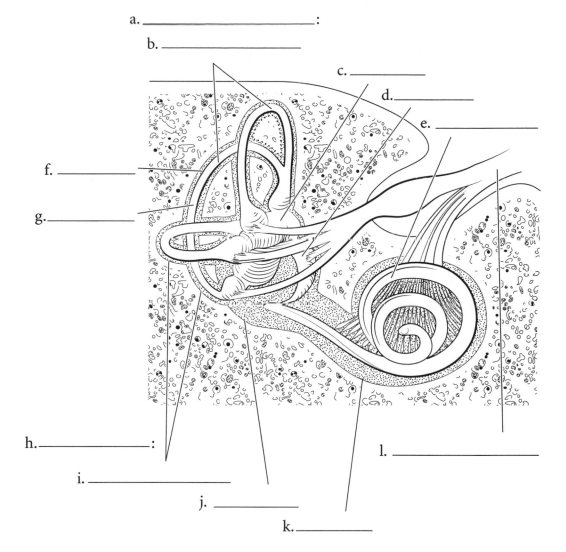

Cross Section of a Semicircular Canal

Look at the cross section of a **semicircular duct**. The outer part of the canal is the **bony labyrinth**. **Perilymph** is the fluid between the bony labyrinth and the **membranous labyrinth**. Inside the membranous labyrinth is a fluid called **endolymph**. Label these structures and fluids.

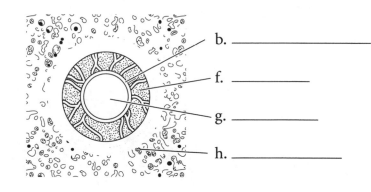

b. _____
f. _____
g. _____
h. _____

Answer Key: a. Membranous labyrinth, b. Semicircular ducts, c. Utricle, d. Saccule, e. Cochlear duct, f. Perilymph, g. Endolymph, h. Bony labyrinth, i. Semicircular canals, j. Vestibule, k. Cochlea, l. Vestibulocochlear nerve

CROSS SECTION OF COCHLEA

Look at the cross section of cochlea. Each coil of the cochlea has three chambers and three membranes. The upper chamber in the illustration is the **scala vestibuli**. It is connected to the oval window. The **vestibular membrane** is the tissue that forms the bottom of the scala vestibuli. Below this is the **scala media** that houses the **spiral organ** (or the **organ of Corti**). The bottom chamber is the **scala tympani**. Between the scala tympani and the scala media is the **basilar membrane**. Label these features and color each space (scala) a different color.

Spiral Organ

The scala media is the region of the cochlea involved in hearing. It is bounded by the **vestibular membrane** on top and the **basilar membrane** on the bottom. Attached to the basilar membrane are the **hair cells**. These cells are attached to the **tectorial membrane** which vibrates when sound impulses enter the cochlea. The tectorial membrane tugs on the hair cells which converts the sound impulse to a neural impulse which travels by the **cochlear nerve** to the brain where hearing is interpreted. Label these structures and color them in, each with a different color.

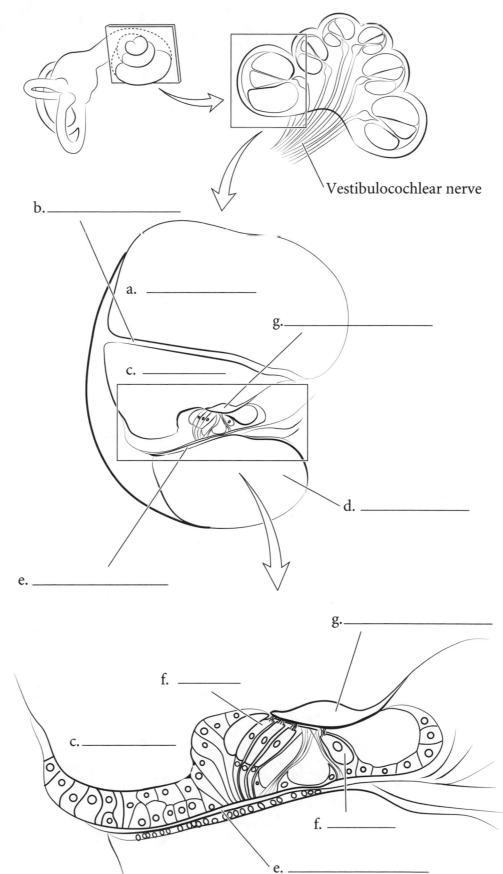

Vestibulocochlear nerve

b. _____

a. _____

g. _____

c. _____

d. _____

e. _____

g. _____

f. _____

c. _____

f. _____

e. _____

Answer Key: a. Scala vestibuli,
b. Vestibular membrane, c. Scala media,
d. Scala tympani, e. Basilar membrane,
f. Hair cell, g. Tectorial membrane

OVERVIEW OF THE ENDOCRINE SYSTEM

The endocrine system is a collection of glands and organs that secrete hormones. This system is grouped according to the function that the individual organs have. Some of these organs have two roles and are called mixed organs. They secrete hormones and also perform other functions such as digestion or secretion. The pancreas is a good example of this. It secretes hormones (an endocrine function) that regulate blood sugar levels and also secretes enzymes (exocrine secretions) that break down material in the digestive tract. Hormones are released from endocrine glands and typically travel through the body in blood vessels and reach target areas that have cells receptive to the hormones. Locate and label the **pineal gland, pituitary gland, thyroid gland, pancreas, adrenal glands, testes,** and **ovaries.** Color the organs in with different colors for each organ.

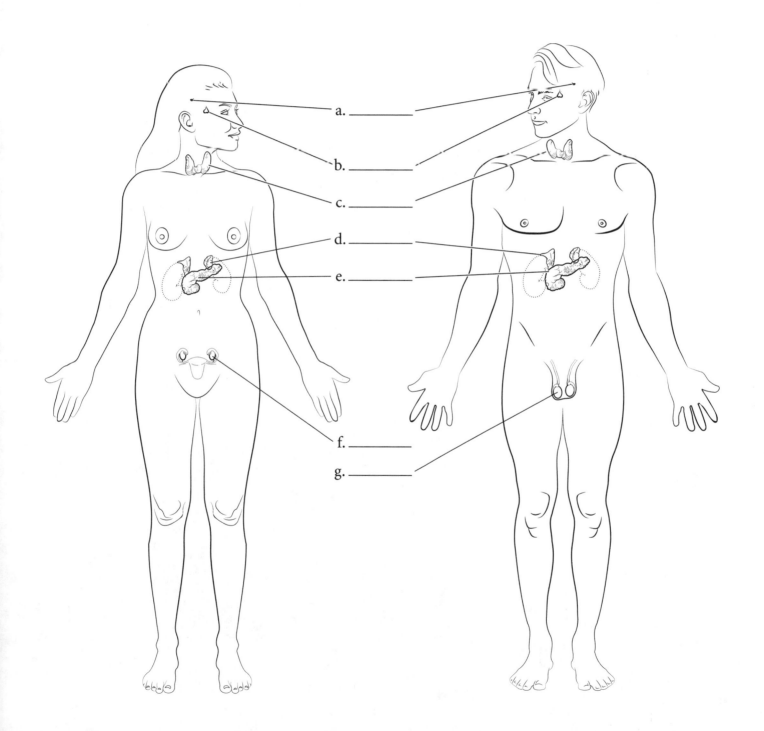

a. _____

b. _____

c. _____

d. _____

e. _____

f. _____

g. _____

Answer Key: a. Pineal gland, b. Pituitary gland, c. Thyroid gland, d. Adrenal glands, e. Pancreas, f. Ovary, g. Testis

ORGANS OF THE HEAD

The **pineal gland** is a small gland located posterior to the **corpus callosum** in the brain. It has the shape of a pine nut but is a little bit smaller. It secretes the hormone melatonin; melatonin levels increase during the night and decrease during the day.

The **pituitary gland**, or **hypophysis**, is suspended from the brain by a stalk called the **infundibulum**. The pituitary sits in the **hypophyseal fossa** which is a depression in the **sphenoid bone**. The pituitary is a complicated gland that has numerous functions. The **adenohypophysis** or **anterior pituitary** originates from the oral cavity during development and consists of epithelium. It produces several hormones which will be discussed later. The anterior pituitary has cells that pick up histological stain differently. These are **acidophilic cells** and **basophilic cells**. The **neurohypophysis** or **posterior pituitary** is derived from the brain during development and does not make its own hormones but stores hormones produced in the hypothalamus. Label the pineal gland, the corpus callosum, and the pituitary gland and color them in. Label the parts of the pituitary and use different colors for each part.

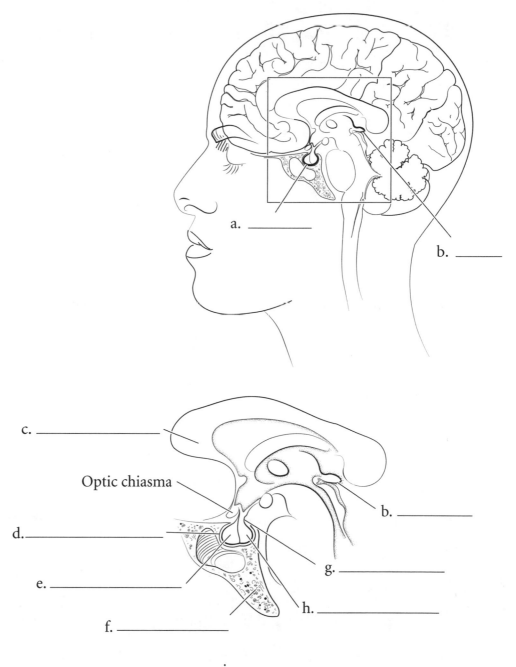

a. _____

b. _____

c. _____

Optic chiasma

b. _____

d. _____

g. _____

e. _____

h. _____

f. _____

i. _____

j. _____

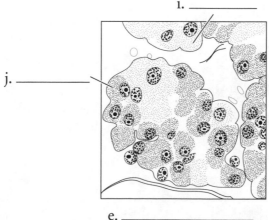
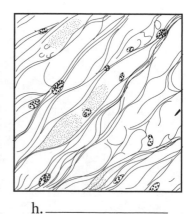

e. _____

h. _____

Answer Key: a. Pituitary gland (hypophysis), b. Pineal gland, c. Corpus callosum, d. Hypophyseal fossa, e. Adenohypophysis (anterior pituitary), f. Sphenoid bone, g. Infundibulum, h. Neurohypophysis (posterior pituitary), i. Basophilic cell j. Acidophilic cell

HORMONES SECRETED BY THE PITUITARY AND THEIR TARGET ORGANS

The **adenohypophysis** produces and secretes many hormones that have diverse target areas. **Growth hormone (GH)** is released by the pituitary and causes growth and division of cells throughout the body. **Prolactin** is more specific in its function. Prolactin stimulates the mammary glands to become functional in milk production. **Follicle stimulating hormone (FSH)** and **luteinizing hormone (LH)** are gonadotropins that cause the ovaries and testes to release hormones. **Thyroid stimulating hormone (TSH)** causes the thyroid gland to secrete hormones and **adrenocorticotropic hormone (ACTH)** has an influence on the adrenal cortex.

The posterior pituitary, or **neurohypophysis**, stores and secretes a hormone called **oxytocin**. This hormone has many functions. It causes milk letdown during nursing and has multiple functions as a neurotransmitter in the brain. It is secreted during orgasm in the female and is also released when the infant is nursing. Oxytocin also has an effect on kidney water balance. The other hormone stored in the neurohypophysis is **antidiuretic hormone** or **ADH**. It is also known as **vasopressin**. It causes absorption of water from the collecting tubules of the kidney decreasing the volume of water in urine.

Answer Key: a. Adenohypophysis, b. Thyroid stimulating hormone, c. Prolactin, d. Growth hormone, e. Adrenocorticotropic hormone, f. Luteinizing hormone, g. Follicle stimulating hormone, h. Neurohypophysis, i. Oxytocin, j. Antidiuretic hormone (vasopressin)

THYROID GLAND

The thyroid gland is just inferior to the thyroid cartilage of the larynx. It has two main **lobes** and a small connection between them called the **isthmus**. The histology of the thyroid is very distinctive. There are cells called **follicular cells** forming a sphere and these make up the follicle. Inside the follicle is the **colloid** where thyroid hormones are stored. The **parafollicular cells** are between the follicles. Label the main parts of the thyroid gland, the follicular cells, the parafollicular cells and the colloid and color them in.

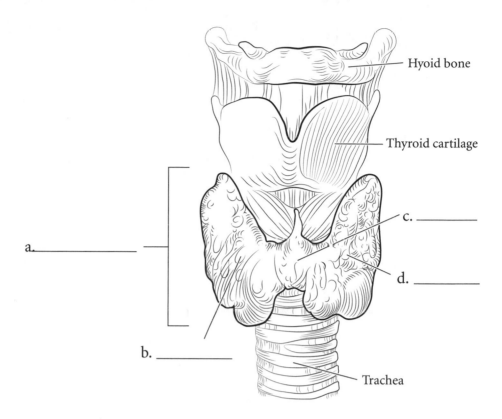

Hyoid bone

Thyroid cartilage

a. _____

c. _____

d. _____

b. _____

Trachea

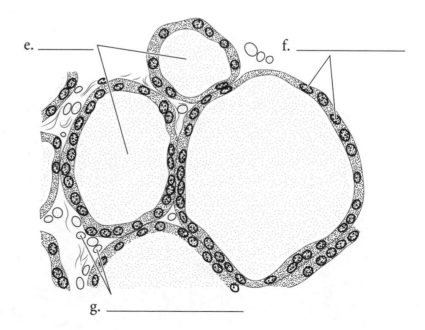

e. _____

f. _____

g. _____

Answer Key: a. Thyroid gland, b. Right lobe, c. Isthmus, d. Left lobe, e. Colloid, f. Follicular cells, g. Parafollicular cells

PARATHYROID GLANDS

There are typically four glands on the posterior of the thyroid gland and these are known as the **parathyroid glands**. They secrete a hormone called parathormone which regulates calcium balance in the blood. Parathormone increases blood calcium levels by causing more absorption of calcium from the digestive tract, increased osteoclast activity in the bones, and reabsorption of calcium from the kidney. The **principal** or **chief cells** secrete parathyroid hormone. The **oxyphilic cells** are less common and their function is poorly understood. Label the parathyroids on the posterior thyroid gland and color them in.

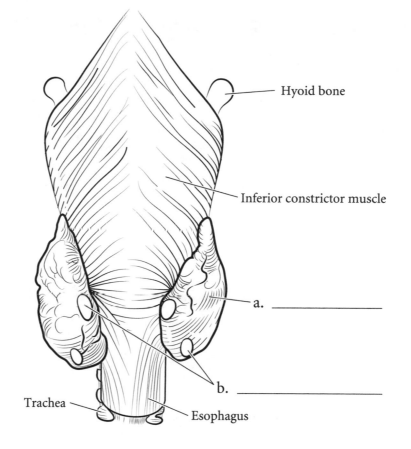

Hyoid bone

Inferior constrictor muscle

a. _____

b. _____

Trachea

Esophagus

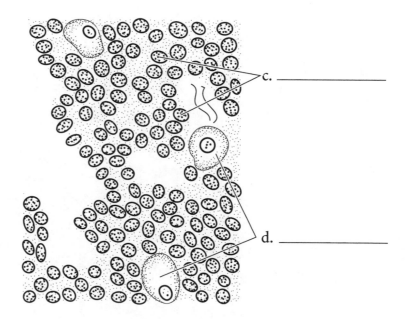

c. _____

d. _____

PANCREAS

The **pancreas** is inferior to the stomach and has several digestive functions. These exocrine secretions are initiated by the **acinar cells**. The endocrine function of the pancreas consists of the secretion of insulin, glucagon, and somatostatin from the **pancreatic islets**. These islets are microscopic collections of cells that have specialized cells for the secretion of hormones. Insulin lowers blood glucose levels while glucagon does the reverse. Somatostatin moderates some of the pancreatic cells that have a role in digestion. Label and color in the pancreas and make the pancreatic islets lighter than the acinar cells of the pancreas.

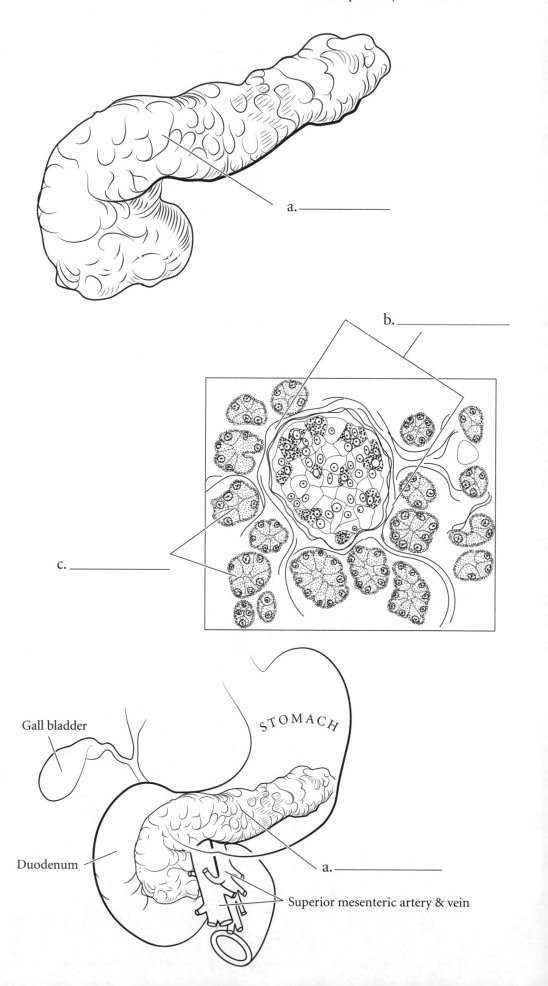

a. _____

b. _____

c. _____

Gall bladder

STOMACH

Duodenum

a. _____

Superior mesenteric artery & vein

Answer Key: a. Pancreas, b. Pancreatic islets, c. Acinar cells (exocrine)

ADRENAL GLANDS

The **adrenal glands** are positioned superior to the kidneys and are divided into the adrenal **cortex** and the **medulla**. The cortex has three layers. The most superficial layer is the **zona glomerulosa**, which is deep to the adrenal capsule and responsible for the secretion of mineralocorticoid hormones. The next layer is the **zona fasciculata** which mainly secretes glucocorticoids, hormones responsible for the breakdown of proteins and lipids and the synthesis of glucose. The **zona reticularis** is the deepest layer of the cortex and it secretes androgens (male sex hormones) and small amounts of estrogens (female sex hormones) in both sexes. The most prevalent male hormone is DHEA (dehydroepiandrosterone) which is responsible for the development of the sex drive, pubic hair, and axillary hair. The effects of DHEA are minimized in males as the testes secrete greater amounts of testosterone. The adrenal medulla is the deepest part of the adrenal gland and it secretes epinephrine and norepinephrine. Label and color the adrenal glands and use a different color for each layer of the cortex and another for the medulla.

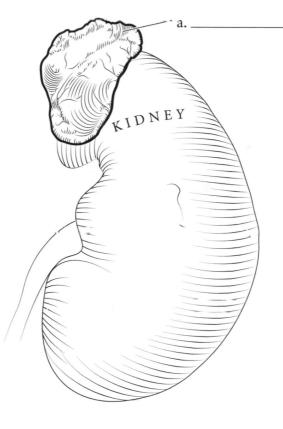

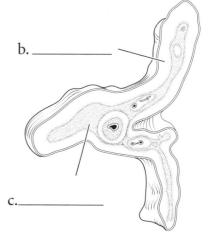

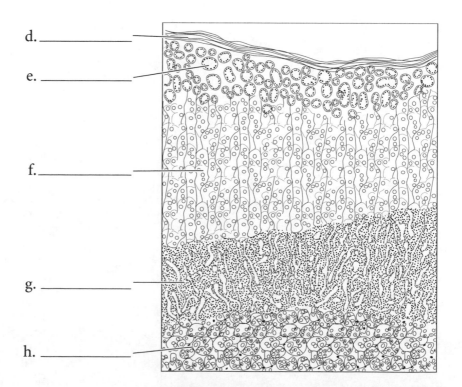

Answer Key: a. Adrenal glands, b. Cortex, c. Medulla, d. Capsule, e. Zona glomerulosa, f. Zona fasciculata, g. Zona reticularis, h. Medulla

GONADS

The **ovaries** are a mixed gland because they produce the oocytes (egg cells) and also have an endocrine function by producing estrogens. Estrogens are a class of female sex hormones that include estradiol and progesterone. Estradiol is produced in the **granulosa cells** of the **ovarian follicles**. These follicles surround the oocytes. Progesterone is produced by the **corpus luteum** after the oocyte has been ovulated.

The **testes** are also mixed glands. As exocrine glands they produce sperm cells and as endocrine glands the **interstitial cells** produce testosterone. Label and color the interstitial cells and **seminiferous tubules** in the microscopic view of the testes.

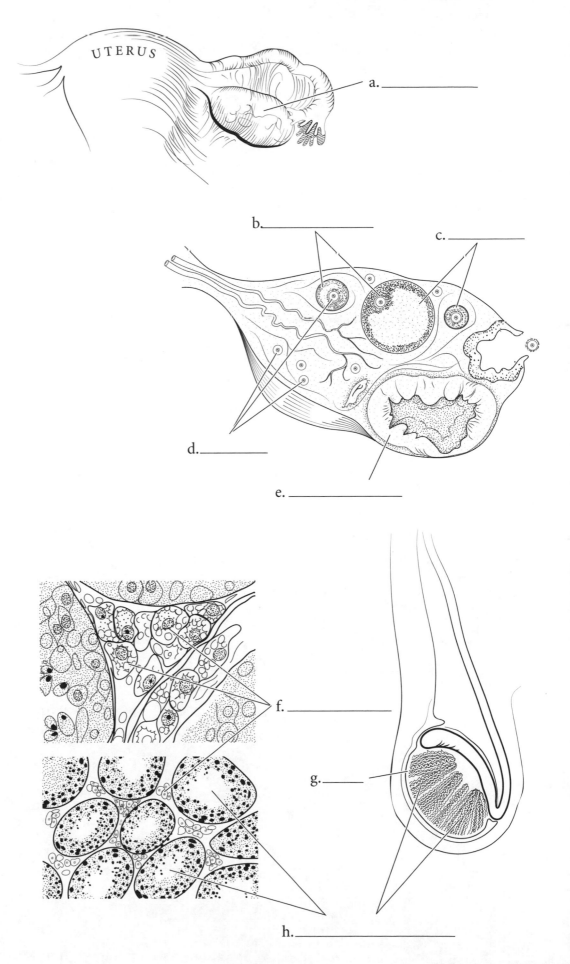

UTERUS

a.

b.

c.

d.

e.

f.

g.

h.

Answer Key: a. Ovary, b. Granulosa cells, c. Ovarian follicles, d. Ova, e. Corpus luteum, f. Interstitial cells, g. Testis, h. Seminiferous tubules

OVERVIEW OF THE CARDIOVASCULAR SYSTEM

The cardiovascular system consists of the heart as a pump, blood vessels that take blood away from the heart (arteries), and blood vessels that take blood back to the heart (veins). Locate the **heart** on the illustration and color it in purple. Label the **common carotid artery** and color it in red. Arteries are typically colored in red and veins are colored blue. Label and color in the **internal jugular vein** too. The internal jugular vein takes blood to the **superior vena cava** which takes blood to the heart. Label and color the **aortic arch** red and find the continuation of the **aorta** that travels down the left side of the body, splits and takes blood to the **femoral artery**. The vessel parallel to the femoral artery is the **femoral vein** and it should be colored blue. The femoral vein takes blood to the **inferior vena cava** before it goes to the heart. Blood travels to the arm by the **brachial artery** and deoxygenated (color it blue) blood travels to the lungs in the **pulmonary trunk**.

a. _____

b. _____

c. _____

d. _____

e. _____

f. _____

g. _____

h. _____

i. _____

j. _____

k. _____

Answer Key: a. Internal jugular vein, b. Common carotid artery, c. Superior vena cava, d. Brachial artery, e. Inferior vena cava, f. Aortic arch, g. Pulmonary trunk, h. Heart, i. Aorta, j. Femoral artery, k. Femoral vein.

CIRCULATION

The heart has four chambers including the superior atria and the inferior ventricles. There is a typical coloring pattern for the cardiovascular system. Vessels or chambers that carry deoxygenated blood are colored in blue while vessels that carry oxygenated blood are colored red. Label and color the **right atrium** (blue), **right ventricle** (blue), **left atrium** (red) and **left ventricle** (red). Remember the heart is in anatomical position so the right atrium is on the left in the illustration.

There are two major circulations in the body. One goes to the lungs and this is called the **pulmonary circulation**. Deoxygenated blood leaves the right ventricle of the heart and travels through the **pulmonary artery** (blue) to the lungs where the blood is oxygenated. Blood returns from the lungs to the left atrium of the heart by the **pulmonary veins** (red). The other main circulation in the body is called the **systemic circulation** where blood travels from the left ventricle of the heart and goes to the other regions of the body. Arteries are vascular tubes that take blood away from the heart while veins are vessels that return blood to the heart. Most arteries carry oxygenated blood and most veins carry deoxygenated blood but there are a few exceptions.

The first vessel that leaves the heart is the **aorta** which is part of the arterial system. Color it red. **Arteries** receive blood from the aorta and take blood throughout the body. They branch and become smaller until they become **arterioles**. The arterioles are the structures that control blood pressure in the body. As they get smaller they become capillaries. The **capillaries** are the site of exchange with the cells of the body. Label and then color the capillaries purple. Purple is a good choice because the capillaries are the interchange between the arteries (red) and the veins (blue). On the return flow the capillaries enlarge and turn into **venules,** which take blood to the veins. Color the venules and remaining **veins** of the body blue. Blood from the inferior portion of the heart returns to the heart by the **inferior vena cava.**

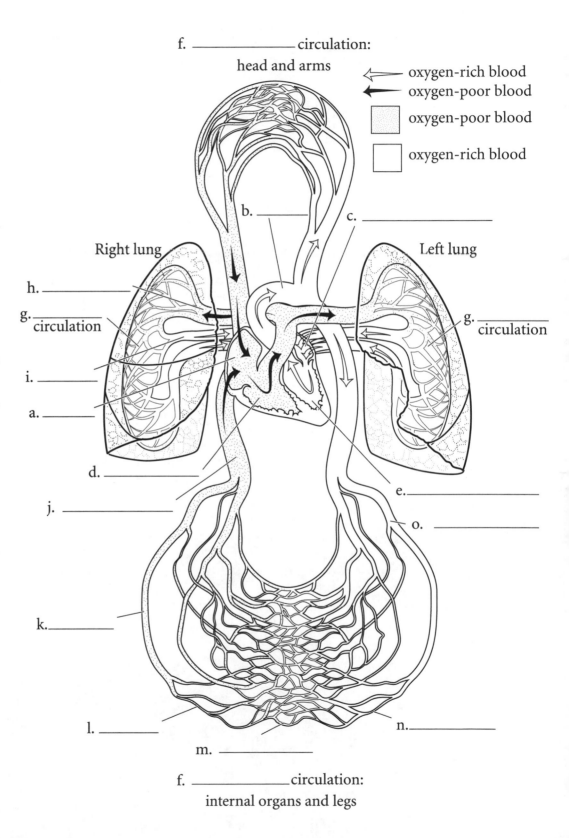

f. _____ circulation: head and arms

→ oxygen-rich blood
→ oxygen-poor blood
▨ oxygen-poor blood
□ oxygen-rich blood

b. _____
c. _____
Right lung
Left lung
h. _____
g. _____ circulation
g. _____ circulation
i. _____
a. _____
d. _____
e. _____
j. _____
o. _____
k. _____
l. _____
n. _____
m. _____
f. _____ circulation: internal organs and legs

Answer Key: a. Right atrium, b. Aorta, c. Left atrium, d. Right ventricle, e. Left ventricle, f. Systemic, g. Pulmonary, h. Pulmonary artery, i. Pulmonary vein, j. Inferior vena cava, k. Vein, l. Venule, m. Capillary, n. Arteriole, o. Artery

BLOOD

Blood consists of **plasma** and **formed elements**. The plasma is the fluid portion of the blood and consists of water, proteins, and dissolved materials such as oxygen, carbon dioxide, electrolytes (ionic particles) and other materials. Plasma makes up about 55% of the blood volume. Formed elements make up about 45% of the blood volume and consist of **erythrocytes** (red blood cells), **leukocytes** (white blood cells) and **thrombocytes** (platelets). Label and color in the red blood cells with a light red color. Label the white blood cells and color in the nucleus with purple and the cytoplasm a light blue. Label and color the thrombocytes purple. There are about 200,00-450,00 thrombocytes per cubic millimeter of blood. They assist the body in clotting to prevent blood from flowing out of small ruptures in blood vessels.

There are about 5 million erythrocytes per cubic millimeter of blood. The erythrocytes do not have a nucleus and they appear like a donut with a thin spot instead of the donut hole. About a third of the weight of a red blood cell is due to **hemoglobin** which makes the cells red. Color in the surface view and cross section of the red blood cell. Note also the size of the thrombocyte.

There are about 7 thousand leukocytes per cubic millimeter of blood. There are two main types of leukocytes; **granular leukocytes** and **agranular leukocytes**. The granular leukocytes have cytoplasmic granules that either stain pink, dark purple or do not stain much at all. The granular leukocytes that do not stain much at all are called **neutrophils** because the granules are neutral to the stains. They are the most numerous of the leukocytes making up 60-70% of the leukocytes. Neutrophils have a three to five lobed nucleus. Color in the cells by shading the cytoplasm light blue and coloring in the nucleus purple.

The **eosinophils** are granular leukocytes that have pink or orange staining granules. The nucleus is generally two-lobed. Color in the eosinophil by first coloring in the purple nucleus and then adding orange to the cytoplasm. Eosinophils make up about 3 percent of the white blood cells.

Basophils are a rare granular leukocyte in that they make up less than one percent of the white blood cells. The nucleus is S-shaped but it is frequently difficult to see because it is obscured by the dark staining cytoplasmic granules. Label the basophil and color in the granules a dark purple.

The two kinds of agranular leukocytes are the **lymphocytes** and the **monocytes**. The lymphocytes can be large or small and they make up 20-30% of the leukocytes. The cytoplasm is light blue and the nucleus is purple. The nucleus of the lymphocyte is dented or flattened. Lymphocytes come in two kinds. **B cells** secrete antibodies (antibody-mediated immunity) and **T cells** which are involved in cell-mediated immunity. Label and color the lymphocytes.

The monocytes are large cells (about 3 times the size of a red blood cell) and they have a strongly lobed nucleus. Some people say this looks like a kidney bean or a horseshoe. They represent only about 5% of the leukocytes. Color in the nucleus with a purple and the cytoplasm a light blue.

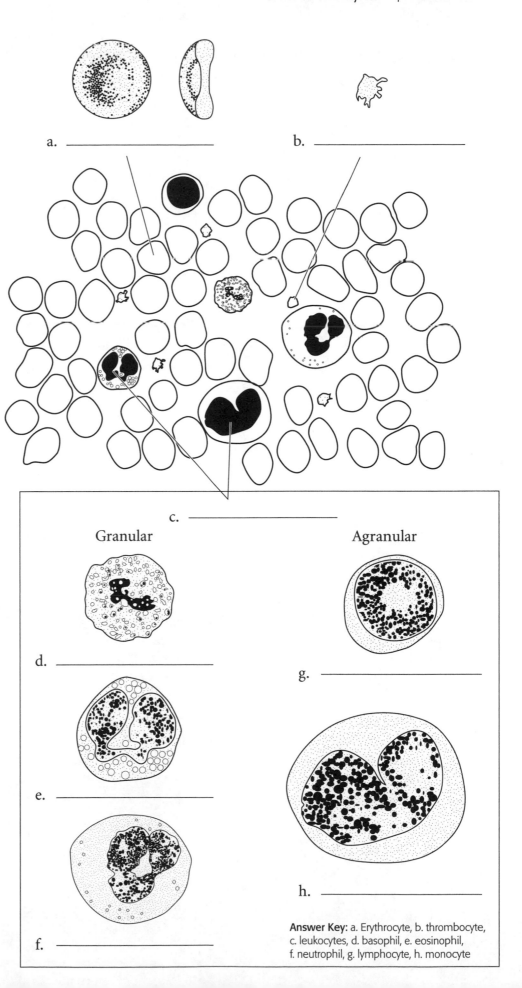

a. _____

b. _____

c. _____

Granular

Agranular

d. _____

g. _____

e. _____

f. _____

h. _____

Answer Key: a. Erythrocyte, b. thrombocyte, c. leukocytes, d. basophil, e. eosinophil, f. neutrophil, g. lymphocyte, h. monocyte

ANTERIOR SURFACE VIEW OF HEART

The **apex** of the heart is inferior and the **base** is superior. Label each chamber of the heart and color them each a different color. Locate the **coronary arteries** and their branches and color them in red. The **right coronary artery** leads to the **right marginal artery**. The **left coronary** artery takes blood to the **anterior interventricular branch** and the **circumflex branch**. The **cardiac veins** can also be seen on the anterior side. The **great cardiac vein** runs in the interventricular sulcus on the anterior side. Label all of the major vessels entering and exiting the heart.

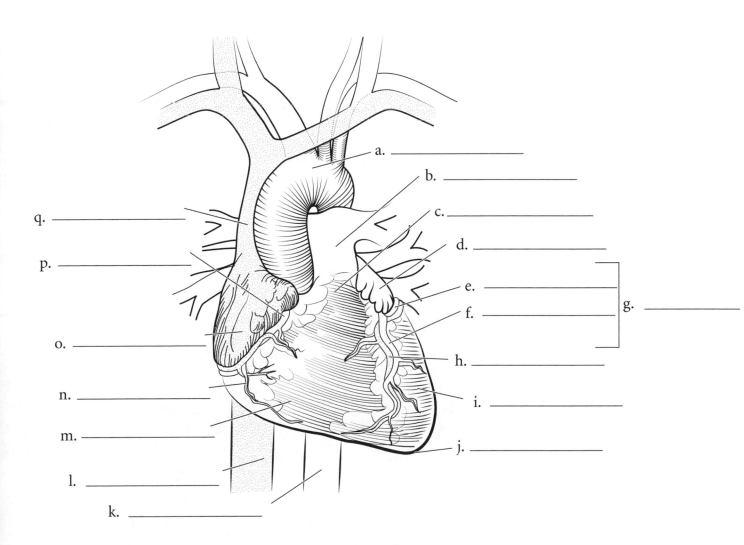

a. _____
b. _____
c. _____
d. _____
e. _____
f. _____
g. _____
h. _____
i. _____
j. _____
k. _____
l. _____
m. _____
n. _____
o. _____
p. _____
q. _____

Answer Key: a. Aortic arch, b. Pulmonary trunk, c. Base of heart, d. Left atrium, e. Circumflex branch, f. Anterior interventricular branch , g. Left coronary artery, h. Great cardiac vein, i. Left ventricle, j. Apex of heart, k. Descending aorta, l. Inferior vena cava, m. Right ventricle, n. Right marginal artery, o. Right atrium, p. Right coronary artery, q. Superior vena cava

POSTERIOR SURFACE OF HEART

On the posterior side of the heart are additional arteries and veins. The **posterior interventricular artery** occurs between the ventricles on the posterior surface. It receives blood from the **right coronary artery**. The **middle cardiac vein** runs the opposite direction and takes blood into the **coronary sinus**. The **small cardiac vein** is also found on the posterior surface of the heart and enters the coronary sinus from the opposite direction. Label the posterior features of the heart and color the arteries in red (except for the **pulmonary arteries** that carry deoxygenated blood—they should be colored in blue). Color the veins in blue (except for the **pulmonary veins** which should be colored in red).

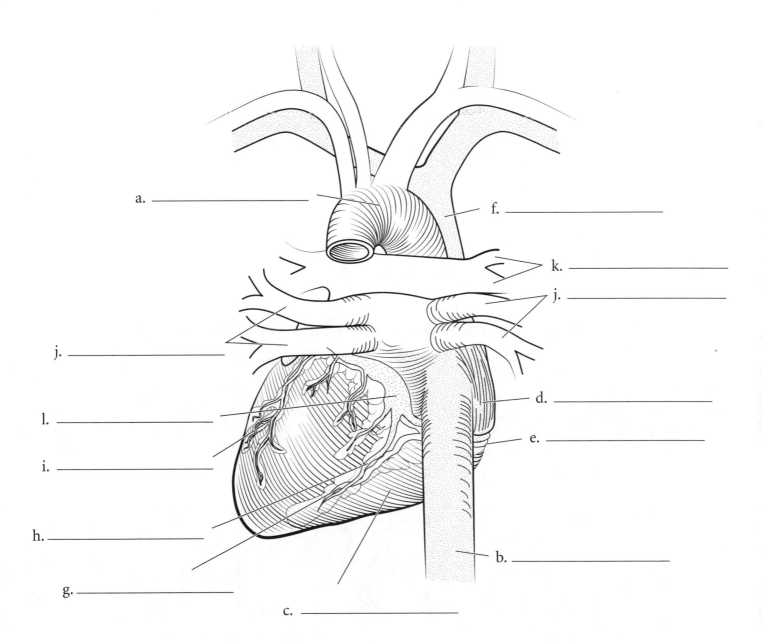

a. _____
f. _____
k. _____
j. _____
j. _____
d. _____
l. _____
e. _____
i. _____
h. _____
b. _____
g. _____
c. _____

Answer Key: a. Aortic arch, b. Inferior vena cava, c. Right ventricle, d. Right atrium, e. Right coronary artery, f. Superior vena cava, g. Posterior interventricular artery, h. Middle cardiac vein, i. Coronary sinus, j. Pulmonary veins, k. Pulmonary arteries, l. Small cardiac vein

CORONAL SECTION OF HEART

The heart is located in a tough, fibrous sac known as the **parietal pericardium** which has an outer **fibrous layer** and an inner **serous layer**. If this sac is opened you can see a space called the pericardial cavity. The heart is in this cavity. The outer surface of the heart is called the **visceral pericardium** or the **epicardium**. Inside of this is the main portion of the heart wall called the **myocardium** (made of cardiac muscle) and the innermost layer of the heart is the **endocardium**.

Deoxygenated blood enters the **right atrium** of the heart by three vessels: the **superior vena cava**, the **inferior vena cava** and the **coronary sinus**. The walls of the right atrium are thin-walled as they only have to pump blood to the **right ventricle**. The blood in the right atrium is in contact with the **fossa ovalis** which is a thin spot in the interatrial septum. This thin spot is a remnant of a hole in the fetal heart know as

the **foramen ovale**. Blood in the right atrium flows through the cusps of the **tricuspid** or **right atrioventricular valve** into the **right ventricle**. The tricuspid valve is made of the three cusps, the **chordae tendineae** and the **papillary muscles** that hold the chordae tendineae to the ventricle wall. The ventricle wall is lined with **trabeculae carneae** that act as struts along the edge of the wall. The wall between the ventricles is known as the **interventricular septum**.

From the right ventricle, blood passes through the **pulmonary semilunar valve** and into the **pulmonary trunk** where the blood goes to the lungs. In the lungs the blood is oxygenated. From the lungs the blood returns to the **left atrium** of the heart. Blood in the left atrium moves to the **left ventricle** through the **left atrioventricular valve** or the **biscuspid valve**. This valve has two cusps, chordae tendineae and papillary muscles. When the left ventricle contracts, the blood moves through the **aortic semilunar valve** and into the **ascending aorta**.

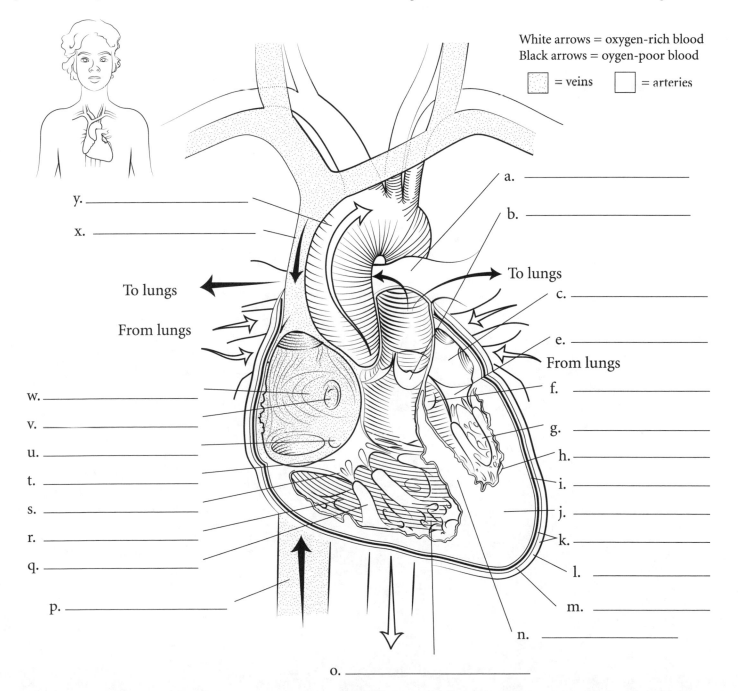

White arrows = oxygen-rich blood
Black arrows = oygen-poor blood

▨ = veins   ☐ = arteries

To lungs

From lungs

To lungs

From lungs

y. _____

x. _____

a. _____

b. _____

c. _____

e. _____

f. _____

g. _____

h. _____

i. _____

j. _____

k. _____

l. _____

m. _____

n. _____

w. _____

v. _____

u. _____

t. _____

s. _____

r. _____

q. _____

p. _____

o. _____

Answer Key: a. Pulmonary trunk, b. Pulmonary semilunar valve, c. Left atrium, e. Left atrioventricular valve, f. Aortric semilunar valve, g. Left ventricle, h. Endocardium, i. Epicardium, j. Myocardium, k. Parietal pericardium, l. Fibrous layer, m. Serous layer, n. Interventricular septum, o. Trabeculae carneae, p. Inferior vena cava, q. Papillary muscle, r. Right ventricle, s. Chordae tendineae, t. Right atrioventricular valve, u. Opening of coronary sinus, v. Fossa ovalis, w. Right atrium, x. Superior vena cava, y. Aorta

SUPERIOR ASPECT OF THE HEART

This view of the heart is seen as if the atria and the major vessels have been removed. You should be able to see all of the major valves of the heart. The most anterior valve is the **pulmonary semilunar valve** that occurs between the right ventricle and the pulmonary trunk. Label and color this valve blue. Posterior to this is the **aortic semilunar valve**. It occurs between the left ventricle and the aorta. Label this valve and color it in red. Both of these valves prevent blood from returning to the ventricles once they have finished contracting. On the right side of the illustration (and on the right side of the heart) is the **right atrioventricular (or tricuspid) valve**, so named because it has three flaps or cusps. This valve occurs between the right atrium and the right ventricle. It prevents the blood from returning to the right atrium during ventricular contraction. Label this valve and color it blue. On the left side of the heart is the **left atrioventricular (bicuspid) valve**. It prevents blood from moving back to the left atrium when the left ventricle contracts.

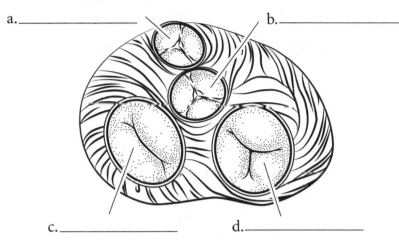

a. _____   b. _____

c. _____   d. _____

ECG—CONDUCTION PATHWAY

The heart has specialized cells that initiate an electrical impulse that radiates throughout the heart. The cells are clustered in a particular area known as the **sinoatrial node** or the pacemaker. These cells produce a depolarization that travels across the atria which depolarize and then contract. Depolarization is an electrical event while contraction is a mechanical event. Between the wall of the right atrium and the right ventricle is a lump of tissue known as the **atrioventricular (AV) node**. Once the impulse reaches this area the AV node pauses a moment before sending the impulse to the **atrioventricular bundle**. This bundle divides into the **bundle branches** and then the impulse travels to the **conduction (Purkinje) fibers**. These fibers reach the muscle of the ventricles and stimulate them to contract. Color each of the components of the conduction pathway a different color.

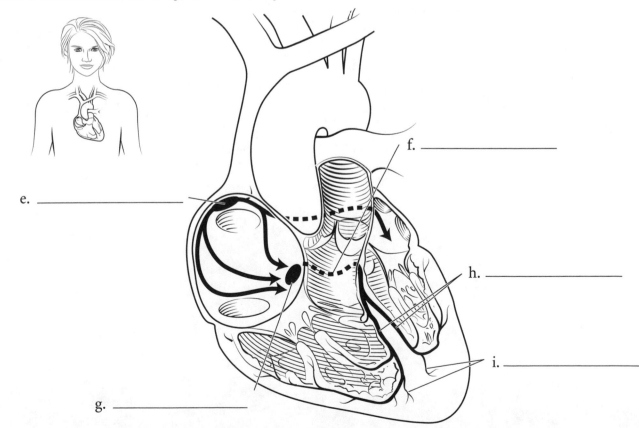

e. _____

f. _____

h. _____

i. _____

g. _____

Answer Key: a. Pulmonary semilunar valve, b. Aortic semilunar valve, c. Left atrioventricular valve, d. Right atrioventricular valve, e. Sinoatrial node, f. Atrioventricular bundle, g. Atrioventricular node, h. Bundle branches, i. Purkinje fibers

VESSELS OVERVIEW

The blood vessels have different thickness due to the differences in pressure that occur in them or their function with respect to exchanging nutrients with the cells. **Arteries** have thick walls due to the higher pressure found in them. Just as high pressure hoses have thick walls so do arteries. The outer layer of the artery is the **tunica externa (tunica adventitia)**. You should locate the tunica externa and color it in. The middle layer of the artery, the **tunica media** is the thickest layer and it is made of **smooth muscle** and **elastic fibers**. Color the tunica media red. The innermost layer of the artery is the **tunica intima (tunica interna)** and it has a special elastic layer called the **lamina elastic interna**. Color this layer. The area in the artery where the blood flows is called the **lumen**.

Veins are thinner walled than arteries and they do not have the same elastic fibers in the tunica media as arteries. Color the tunica media of the veins red and select the same colors as you did for the arteries for the tunica externa and the tunica interna. The tunica interna of veins is folded into valves that allow for a one-way flow of blood through veins.

Capillaries are different from both arteries and veins in that they are composed of only simple squamous epithelium (called **endothelium**). The thin nature of capillaries allows them to exchange nutrients, water, carbon dioxide and oxygen with the cells. Color in the endothelium of the capillary with the same color that you selected for the tunica interna.

Answer Key: a. Vein, b. Artery, c. Lumen, d. Tunica intima, e. Tunica media, f. Tunica externa, g. Lamina elastica interna, h. Lamina elastica externa, i. Smooth muscle, j. Venule, k. Endothelium, l. Arteriole, m. Capillary, n. Venous valve

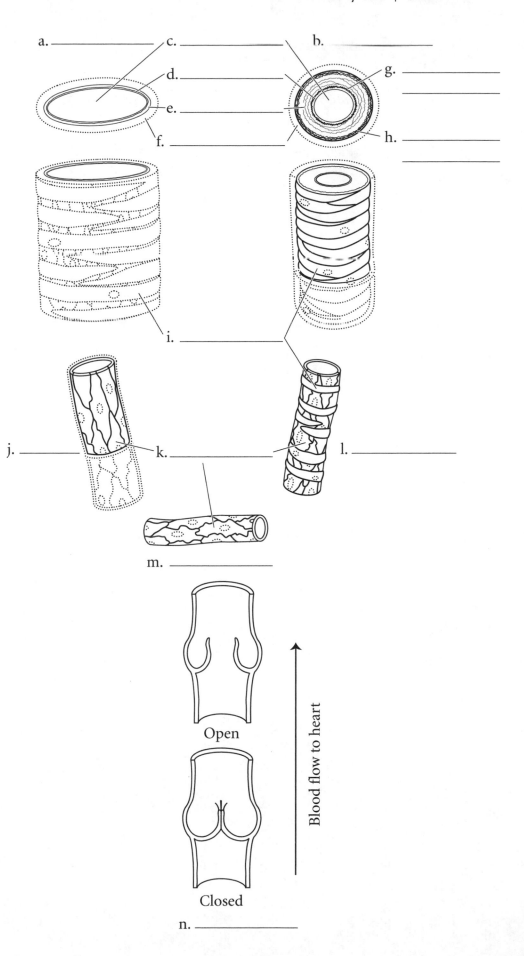

ARTERY OVERVIEW

One of the ways to study arteries is to draw them as if you were making a street map. Begin with the heart and draw the blood vessels that occur as you take blood to the fingers, toes or to a particular organ of the body. Arteries are typically colored red and you should select that color for this illustration. Use the following artery list and label the appropriate arteries and color them in red. The abbreviation for artery is *a*.

Ascending aorta
Aortic arch
Thoracic aorta
Abdominal aorta
Brachiocephalic trunk
Common carotid artery
Subclavian artery
Axillary artery
Brachial artery
Radial artery
Ulnar artery
Common iliac artery
Femoral artery
Anterior tibial artery
Fibular artery

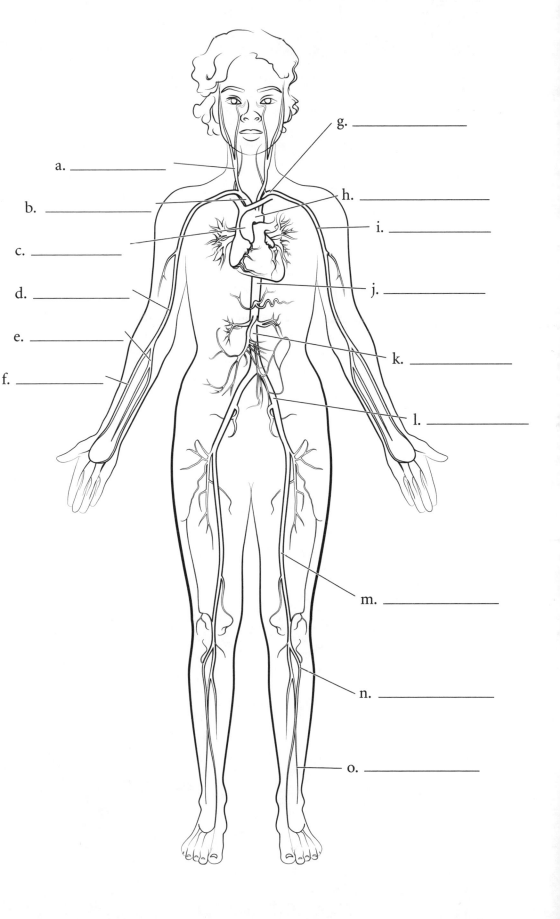

a. _____
b. _____
c. _____
d. _____
e. _____
f. _____
g. _____
h. _____
i. _____
j. _____
k. _____
l. _____
m. _____
n. _____
o. _____

Answer Key: a. Common carotid a., b. Brachiocephalic trunk, c. Ascending aorta, d. Brachial a., e. Ulnar a., f. Radial a., g. Subclavian a., h. Aortic arch, i. Axillary a., j. Thoracic aorta, k. Abdominal aorta, l. Common iliac a., m. Femoral a., n. Anterior tibial a., o. Fibular a.

HEAD AND AORTIC ARTERIES

Blood from the heart exits the **brachiocephalic artery** and takes two main pathways to the right side of the head. One of these is the **right common carotid artery** which exits the brachiocephalic artery and then splits into the **external carotid artery** and the **internal carotid artery**. The external carotid artery has several branches, among them the **facial artery**, the **superficial temporal artery**, the **maxillary artery**, and the **occipital artery**. The internal carotid artery takes blood through the carotid canal of the skull and into the brain. The other main pathway of blood to the right side of the head is the **vertebral artery** which arises from the **subclavian artery**. The left side of the head has a similar pathway except that the **left common carotid artery** and the **left subclavian artery** arise from the aortic arch and not from the brachiocephalic artery. Label these vessels and color them in red.

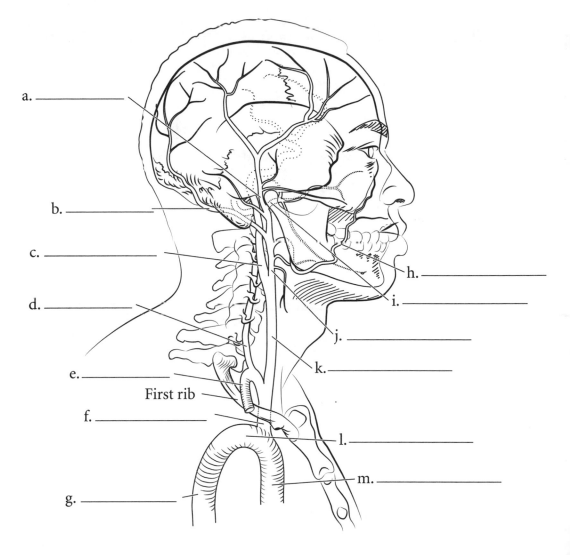

First rib

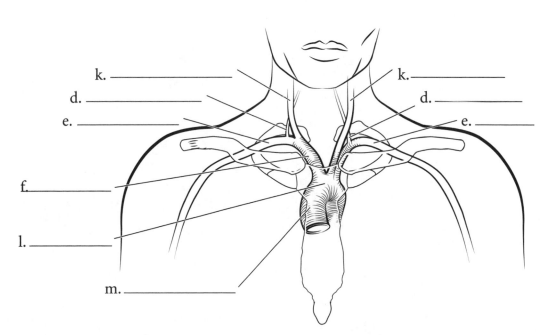

Answer Key: a. Superficial temporal a., b. Occipital a., c. Internal carotid a., d. Vertebral a., e. Subclavian a., f. Brachiocephalic a., g. Thoracic aorta, h. Facial a., i. Maxillary a., j. External carotid a., k. Common carotid a., l. Aortic arch, m. Ascending aorta

BRAIN ARTERIES

The brain is nourished by two main arterial conduits. The first of these is the flow from the **internal carotid arteries**. Blood from the internal carotid arteries comes from the neck and enters a circular pathway known as the **arterial circle** (**circle of Willis**). The other conduit comes from the vertebra and these are the **vertebral arteries**. These arteries connect at a vessel called the **basilar artery** and it leads to the arterial circle. The arterial circle consists of the **anterior communicating arteries** and the **posterior communicating arteries**. From this circle blood then moves into one of many arteries that feed the brain. The cerebrum is fed by the **anterior**, **middle** and **posterior cerebral arteries**. The cerebellum is fed by the **cerebellar arteries**. If there is a blockage in any of these vessels then blood does not reach the affected part of the brain and this produces a stroke. Color the arteries red and label the illustration. Arteries are abbreviated *aa*.

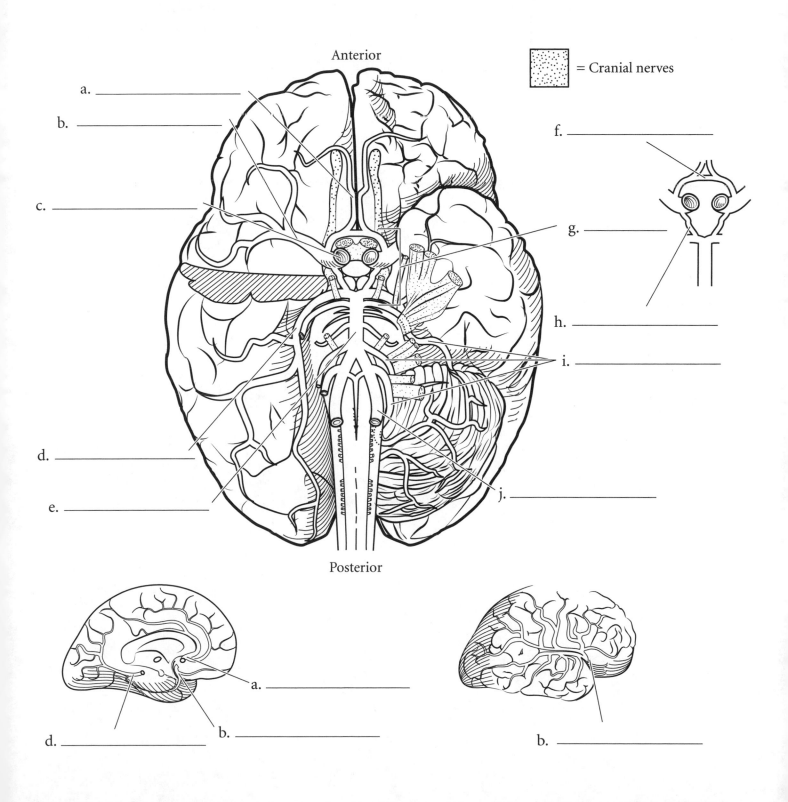

Anterior

= Cranial nerves

a. _____

b. _____

c. _____

d. _____

e. _____

f. _____

g. _____

h. _____

i. _____

j. _____

Posterior

a. _____

d. _____

b. _____

b. _____

Answer Key: a. Anterior cerebral a., b. Middle cerebral a., c. Internal carotid a., d. Posterior cerebral a., e. Basilar a., f. Anterior communicating a., g. Arterial circle, h. Posterior communicating a., i. Cerebellar aa., j. Vertebral a.

UPPER LIMB ARTERIES

The arteries of the upper limb receive blood from the **subclavian artery** which takes blood to the **axillary artery**. Blood in the axillary artery travels to the anterior scapula by the **subscapular artery**, to the external chest wall by the **lateral thoracic artery**, to the upper humeral region by the **posterior circumflex humeral artery**, and to the distal regions of the arm by the **brachial artery**. The brachial artery is the major artery of the arm and it divides distally to form the **radial and ulnar arteries**. The radial artery is frequently palpated at the wrist to determine the pulse rate. The radial and ulnar arteries rejoin (called collateral circulation) in the hand as the **superficial** and **deep palmar arch arteries**. These arteries take blood to the fingers as **digital arteries**. Label these blood vessels and color them red.

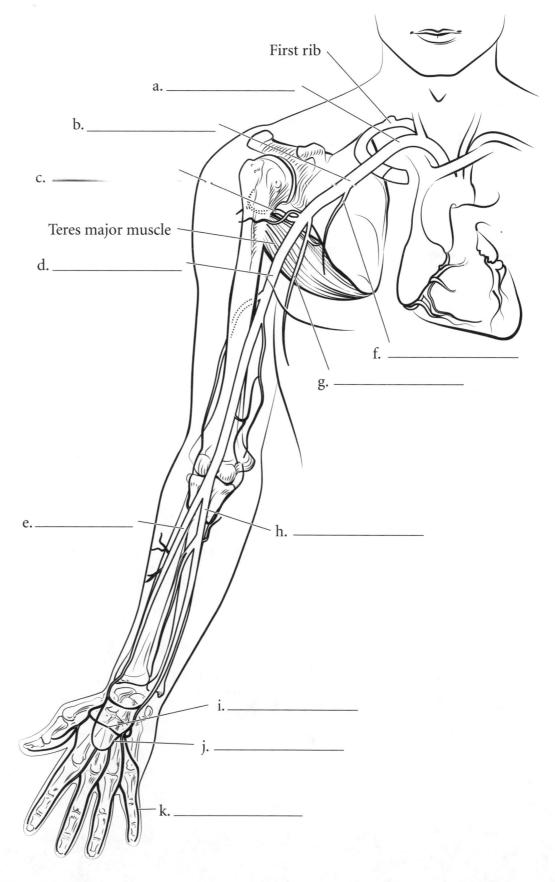

First rib

a. _____

b. _____

c. _____

Teres major muscle _____

d. _____

f. _____

g. _____

e. _____

h. _____

i. _____

j. _____

k. _____

Answer Key: a. Subclavian a., b. Axillary a., c. Posterior circumflex humeral a., d. Brachial a., e. Radial a., f. Lateral thoracic a., g. Subscapular a. , h. Ulnar a., i. Deep palmar arch, j. Superficial palmar arch, k. Digital a.

LOWER LIMB ARTERIES

Blood in the lower limb comes from the branches of the iliac arteries. Blood in the **common iliac artery** flows into the **internal iliac artery** and into the **external iliac artery**. Once it passes by the inguinal ligament (a connective tissue band that stretches from the ilium to the pubis) the external iliac artery becomes the **femoral artery**. The femoral artery takes blood down the anterior thigh but there is a branch called the **deep femoral artery** that takes blood closer to the bone. The femoral artery moves posteriorly to become the **popliteal artery** and branches of the popliteal artery become the **anterior** and **posterior tibial arteries** and the **peroneal (fibular) artery**. The tibial arteries take blood to the **dorsal arcuate artery**, the **dorsalis pedis artery**, and the **dorsal metatarsal arteries** which take blood to the **digital arteries**. Label the lower limb arteries and color them in red.

a. _____

b. _____

c. _____

d. _____

e. _____

f. _____

g. _____

h. _____

i. _____

j. _____

k. _____

l. _____

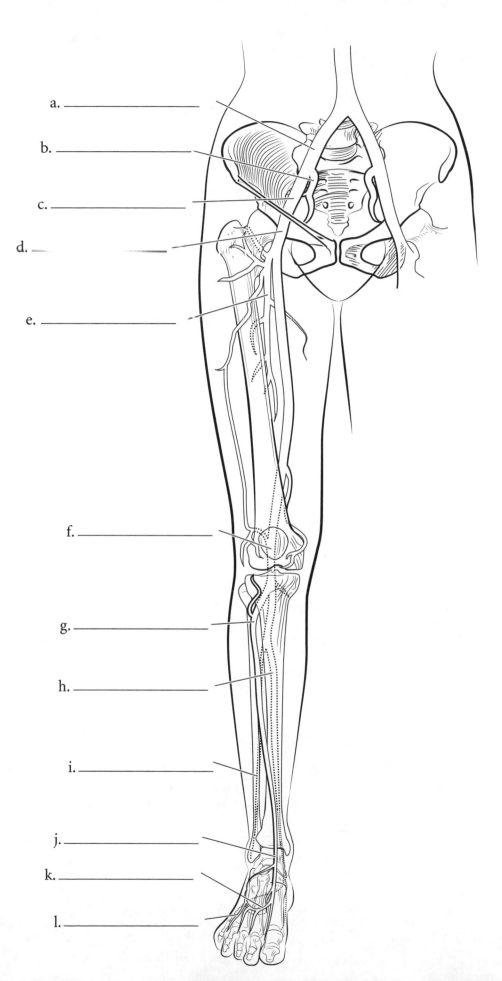

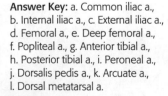

Answer Key: a. Common iliac a., b. Internal iliac a., c. External iliac a., d. Femoral a., e. Deep femoral a., f. Popliteal a., g. Anterior tibial a., h. Posterior tibial a., i. Peroneal a., j. Dorsalis pedis a., k. Arcuate a., l. Dorsal metatarsal a.

ABDOMINAL/THORACIC ARTERIES

The aorta starts at the **ascending aorta** and curves via the **aortic arch**. The **thoracic aorta** is a portion of the descending aorta. It has several branches that take blood to most of the ribs and intercostal muscles. These are the **posterior intercostal arteries**. Below the diaphragm the descending aorta is known as the **abdominal aorta** and it has several branches. The first of these is the **celiac trunk** and it branches to take blood to the stomach, spleen and liver. The next branch is the **superior mesenteric artery**. Below this are the **renal arteries** that take blood to the kidneys. The **gonadal arteries** are found inferior to the renal arteries and they take blood to the testes in males or the ovaries in females. A single **inferior mesenteric artery** is found below the gonadal arteries. The aorta terminates as it divides into the **common iliac arteries**. Label these vessels and color them in red.

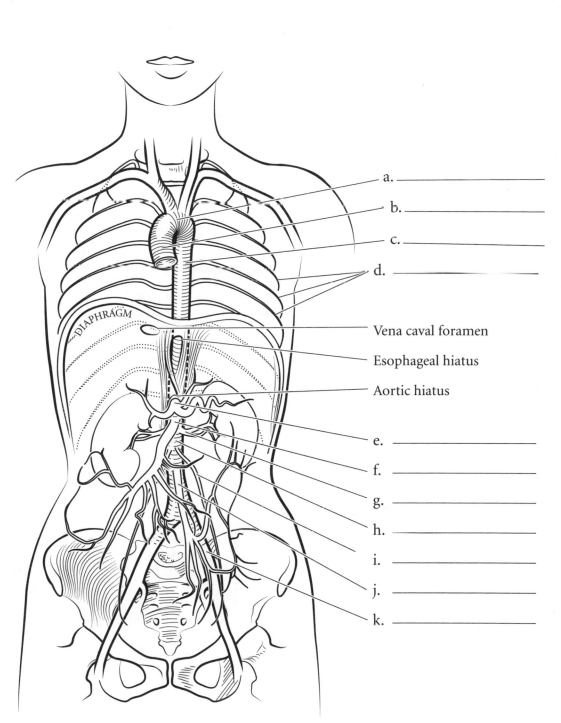

a. _____

b. _____

c. _____

d. _____

Vena caval foramen

Esophageal hiatus

Aortic hiatus

e. _____

f. _____

g. _____

h. _____

i. _____

j. _____

k. _____

DIAPHRÁGM

Answer Key: a. Aortic arch,
b. Ascending aorta, c. Thoracic aorta,
d. Posterior intercostal arteries, e. Celiac trunk, f. Superior mesenteric artery,
g. Renal artery, h. Abdominal aorta,
i. Gonadal artery, j. Inferior mesenteric artery, k . Common iliac artery

ARTERIES OF DIGESTIVE SYSTEM

The **celiac trunk** splits into three branches, the **common hepatic artery**, the left **gastric artery** and the **splenic artery**. There are other branches to the stomach which have collateral circulation (two or more arteries taking blood to one area). One of these is the **right gastroepiploic artery** and another is the **left gastroepiploic artery**. Below the celiac trunk is the **superior mesenteric artery** which takes blood to the small intestine and to several of the colic arteries that supply blood to the proximal portion of the large intestine. These are the **middle colic artery**, the **intestinal branches**, the **right colic artery** and the **ileocolic artery**. The **inferior mesenteric artery** takes blood to the distal portion of the large intestine via the **left colic artery**, **sigmoid artery** and the **rectal artery**.

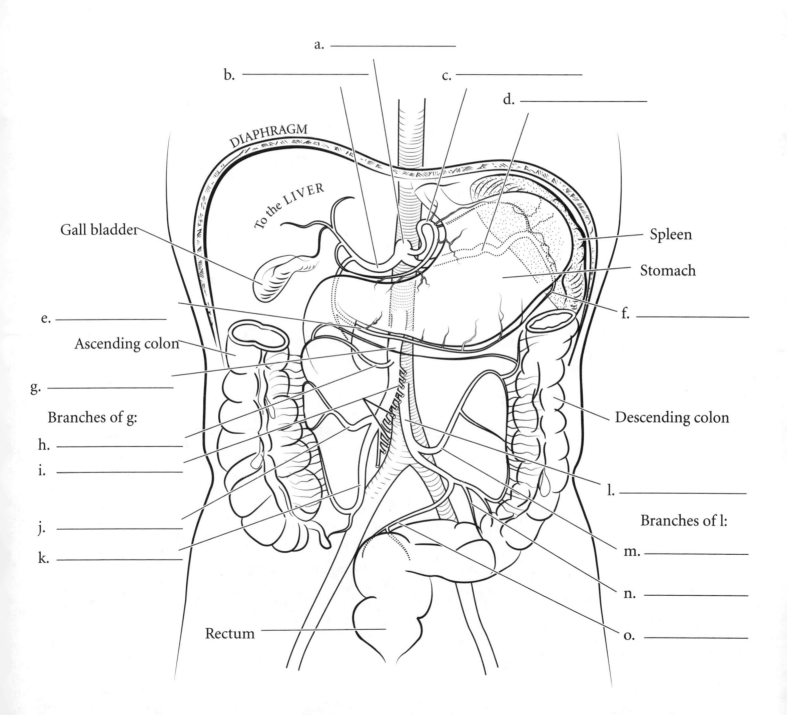

Answer Key: a. Celiac trunk, b. Common hepatic a., c. Left gastric a., d. Splenic a., e. Right gastroepiploic a., f. Left gastroepiploic a., g. Superior mesenteric a., h. Middle colic a., i. Intestinal branches, j. Right colic a., k. Ileocolic a., l. Inferior mesenteric a., m. Left colic a., n. Sigmoid a., o. Superior rectal a.

MALE AND FEMALE PELVIC ARTERIES

The **common iliac artery** takes blood to the **external iliac artery** and the **internal iliac artery** that takes blood to the pelvis. In females, branches of the internal iliac artery take blood to the inner pelvis. The **vesical arteries** takes blood to the bladder, the **uterine arteries** take blood to the uterus, the **vaginal arteries** feed the vagina, the **rectal arteries** feed the rectum, and the sacral arteries go to the sacrum. The **pudendal artery** takes blood to the external regions where it supplies blood to the pelvic floor, the labia majora and minora and the clitoris.

In males the internal iliac artery takes blood to the bladder, rectum, sacrum, the prostate, and seminal vesicles on the inside. The pudendal artery takes blood to the scrotum, penis and external pelvic floor. In both sexes the **obturator artery** takes blood from the internal iliac artery to the medial thigh while the **gluteal arteries** take blood to the muscles posterior to the pelvic cavity.

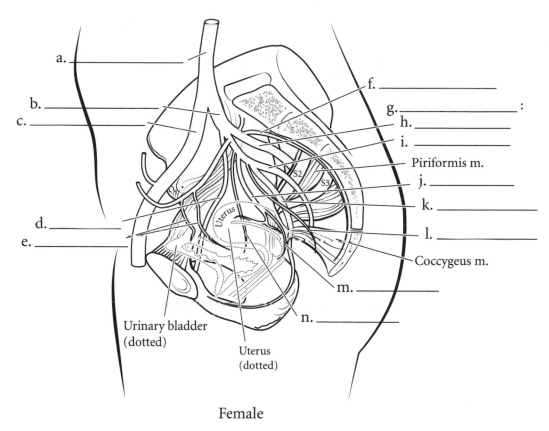

Female

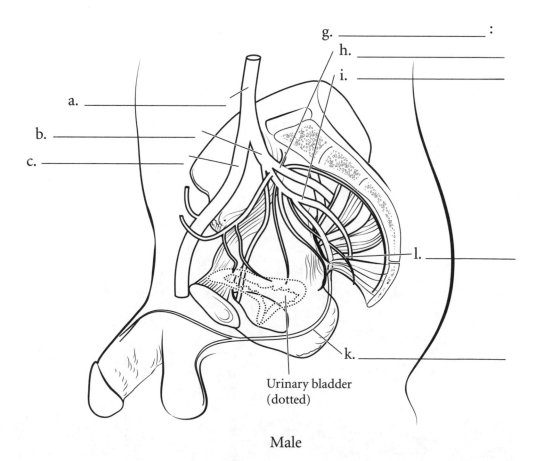

Male

Answer Key: a. Common iliac a., b. Internal iliac a., c. External iliac a., d. Obturator a., e. Superior vesical aa., f. Lateral sacral a., g. Gluteal aa., h. Superior gluteal a., i. Inferior gluteal a., j. Uterine a., k. Pudendal a., l. Middle rectal a., m. Vaginal a., n. Inferior vesical a.

VEINS

Veins are blood vessels that return blood to the heart. They are characteristically colored in blue on illustrations. The deep veins typically take the name of the artery next to them or the name of the organ that provides them with blood. Therefore the femoral vein runs next to the femoral artery and the splenic vein receives blood from the spleen. Some veins have names unique to them and these are typically the superficial veins. Use the following list and label the major veins of the body and color them blue.

Cephalic vein
Basilic vein
Radial veins
Ulnar veins
Brachial vein
Axillary vein
Subclavian vein
Brachiocephalic vein
Superior vena cava
Vertebral vein
Internal jugular vein
External jugular vein
Femoral vein
Great saphenous vein
Small saphenous vein
External iliac vein
Internal iliac vein
Common iliac vein
Inferior vena cava
Renal veins
Gonadal veins

a. _____
b. _____
c. _____

j. _____
k. _____
l. _____
m. _____

Superficial veins:
n. _____
o. _____
p. _____
q. _____
r. _____
s. _____

Deep veins:
d. _____
e. _____
f. _____
g. _____
h. _____

Deep vein:
i. _____

Superficial veins:
t. _____
u. _____

Answer Key: a. Internal jugular vein, b. Brachiocephalic vein, c. Superior vena cava, d. Brachial veins, e. Ulnar veins, f. Radial veins, g. Internal iliac vein, h. External iliac vein, i. Femoral vein, j. Vertebral vein, k. External jugular vein, l. Subclavian vein, m. Axillary vein, n. Cephalic vein, o. Basilic vein, p. Inferior vena cava, q. Renal vein, r. Gonadal vein, s. Common iliac vein, t. Great saphenous vein, u. Small saphenous vein

HEAD/NECK VEINS

Superior Vena Cava Veins

The drainage of the head occurs by the **jugular veins** or the **vertebral veins**. Some of the blood coming from the brain travels down the **superior sagittal sinus** and through the large **internal jugular veins**. These veins take blood down both sides of the neck and enter the

brachiocephalic veins. The external portion of the head is drained by several veins. The **facial vein** and the **maxillary vein** take blood to the internal jugular vein while the **superficial temporal vein** and the **posterior auricular vein** take blood to the **external jugular vein** which then flows into the subclavian vein before reaching the brachiocephalic vein.

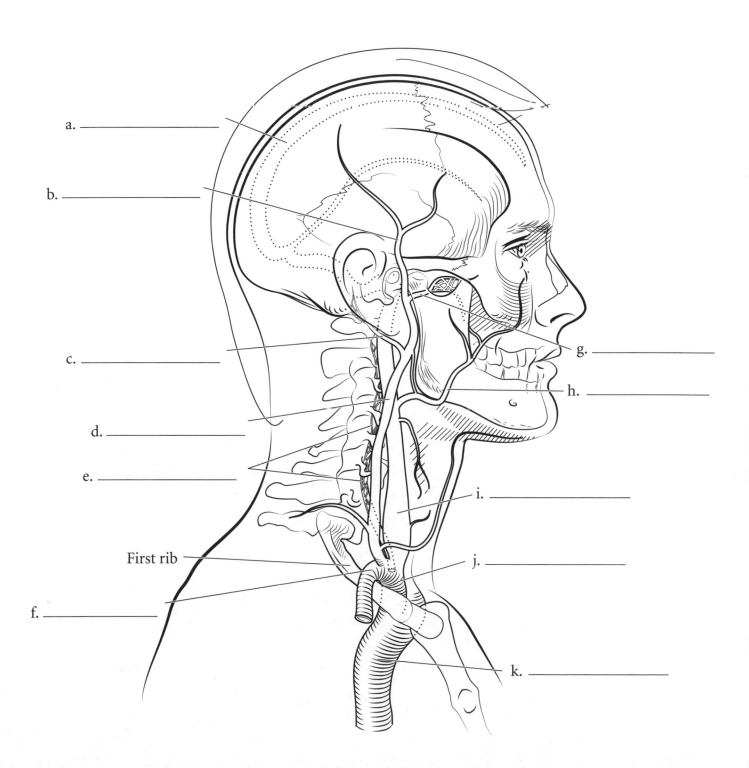

a. _____

b. _____

c. _____

d. _____

e. _____

First rib _____

f. _____

g. _____

h. _____

i. _____

j. _____

k. _____

Answer Key: a. Sagittal sinus, b. Superficial temporal v., c. Posterior auricular v., d. External jugular v., e. Vertebral v. (plexus), f. Subclavian v., g. Maxillary v., h. Facial v., i. Internal jugular v., j. Brachiocephalic v., k. Superior vena cava

UPPER LIMB VEINS

The veins of the upper limb are somewhat variable and have many cross connections between them but they can be divided into the deep veins and the superficial veins. The deep veins of the upper limb frequently form a meshwork around the arteries (venae comitantes) which allows for a great amount of heat transfer. Cool blood from the extremities is warmed by the arterial blood flowing in a counter current. Blood in the fingers returns to the forearm by the **digital veins** and then the **superficial** and **deep palmar arch veins**. The deep veins of the upper limb are the **radial veins**, the **ulnar veins**, and the **brachial veins**. The **brachial** veins lead to the **axillary vein** which takes blood to the **subclavian vein**. The superficial veins of the upper limb are the **basilic vein**, found on the medial aspect of the forearm and arm, the **median antebrachial vein**, on the anterior aspect of the forearm, the **cephalic vein**, found on the lateral aspect of the forearm and arm and a small vein that connects the basilic vein with the cephalic vein called the **median cubital vein**. This vein is used frequently to withdraw blood. Label the veins of the upper limb and color them in blue.

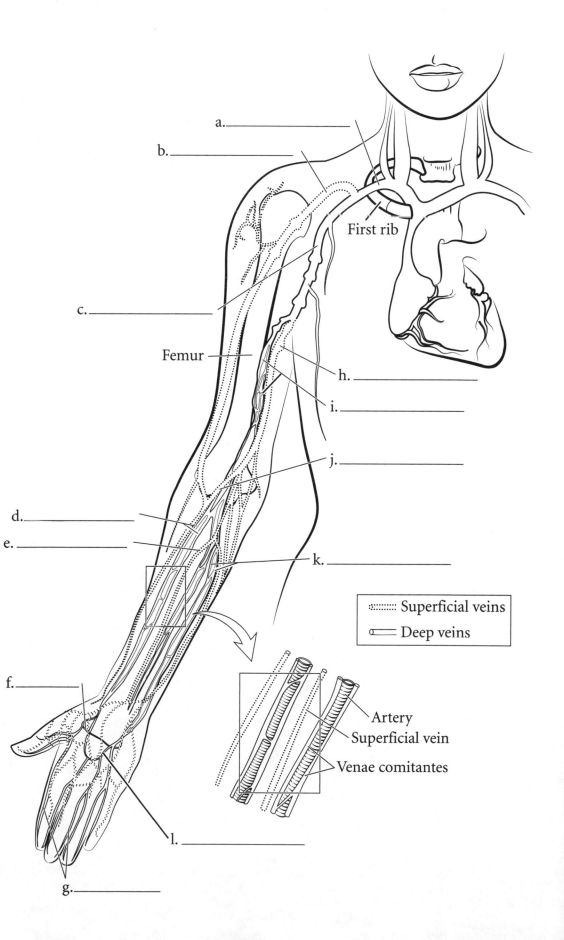

a. _____

b. _____

First rib

c. _____

Femur

h. _____

i. _____

j. _____

d. _____

e. _____

k. _____

⫶⫶⫶⫶ Superficial veins
▭ Deep veins

f. _____

Artery
Superficial vein
Venae comitantes

l. _____

g. _____

Answer Key: a. Subclavian v.,
b. Cephalic v., c. Axillary v., d. Radial vv.,
e. Median antebrachial v., f. Deep palmar arch, g. Digital vv., h. Basilic v.,
i. Brachial vv., j. Median cubital v.,
k. Ulnar vv., l. Superficial palmar arch v.

LOWER LIMB VEINS

Blood in the toes returns by the **digital veins**. These veins take blood to the **dorsal metatarsal veins** and the **dorsal venous arch veins**. On the underside of the foot are the **plantar veins**. Blood moves up the leg by the **posterior** and **anterior tibial veins** and the **great** and **small saphenous veins**. The **anterior** and **posterior tibial veins** join together to form the **popliteal vein** posterior to the knee. The small saphenous vein joins the **popliteal vein** taking blood to the **femoral vein**. The **great saphenous vein** begins around the medial malleolus and runs the entire length of the medial lower limb when it enters into the femoral veins. Once the femoral vein crosses the inguinal ligament it becomes the **external iliac vein**.

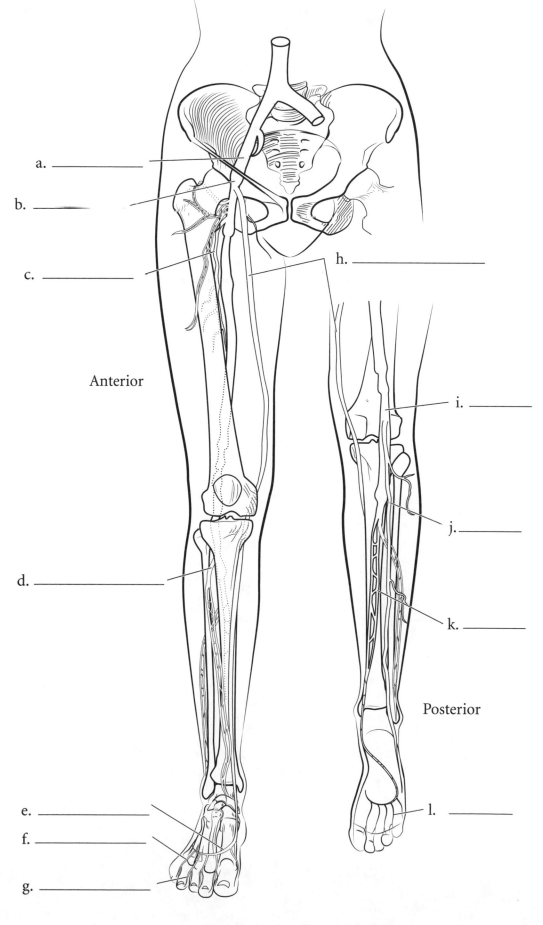

Anterior

Posterior

Answer Key: a. External iliac v., b. Femoral v., c. Deep femoral v., d. Anterior tibial v., e. Dorsal venous arch, f. Dorsal metatarsal v., g. Digital v., h. Great saphenous v., i. Popliteal v., j. Small saphenous v., k. Posterior tibial v., l. Plantar v.

HEPATIC PORTAL VEINS, TRUNK VEINS

Most of the blood of the body returns to the heart by capillaries flowing into venules and finally into veins before reaching the heart. In a **portal system** blood moves from one capillary system to another capillary system before reaching the heart. The **hepatic portal system** takes blood from the capillary beds of many of the abdominal organs and carries it to the liver where metabolic processing takes place. The **hepatic portal vein** receives blood from various veins including the **splenic vein**, the **gastroepiploic vein**, the **left gastric vein** and the **colic veins** which take blood to the **superior mesenteric** and **inferior mesenteric veins**. Once the blood is processed in the liver it enters the systemic circulation by the **hepatic veins**.

The return of blood from other parts of the pelvic and abdominal cavities does not go through the hepatic portal system but enters the inferior vena cava. The **renal veins** take blood from the kidneys to the inferior vena cava. The **gonadal veins** take blood from the testes or the ovaries. The **left gonadal vein** enters **the left renal vein** while the **right gonadal vein** enters the **inferior vena cava**. The **intercostal veins** take blood to the **hemiazygos** and the **azygos veins**.

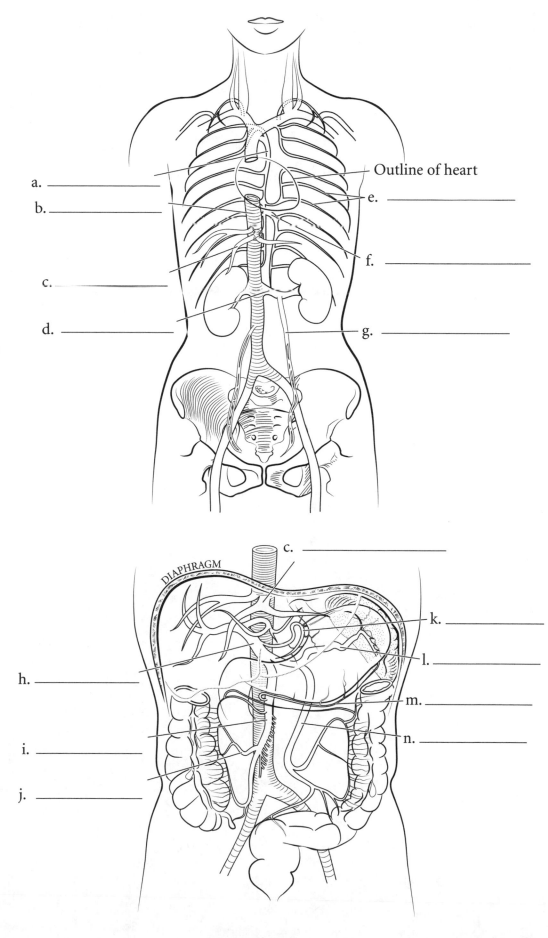

Outline of heart

a. _____
b. _____
c. _____
d. _____
e. _____
f. _____
g. _____

DIAPHRAGM

c. _____
h. _____
i. _____
j. _____
k. _____
l. _____
m. _____
n. _____

Answer Key: a. Azygos v., b. Inferior vena cava, c. Hepatic vv, d. Renal v., e. Posterior intercostal vv., f. Hemiazygos v., g. Gonadal v., h. Hepatic portal v., i. Superior mesenteric v., j. Right colic v., k. Gastric v., l. Splenic v., m. Gastroepiploic v., n. Inferior mesenteric v.

FETAL CIRCULATION

The significant difference in fetal circulation from adult circulation lies in the fact that the lungs are non-functional in the fetus. The source of oxygen for the fetus is the **placenta** where maternal blood carries oxygen and nutrients to the fetus. Blood from the placenta travels to the fetus by the **umbilical vein**. It is called a vein because it carries blood to the fetal heart. The blood flowing in the umbilical vein is oxygenated blood which is not typical of most blood that occurs in veins. From the umbilical vein the blood passes through a small shunt vessel known as the **ductus venosus** and enters the **inferior vena cava** where it mixes with blood returning from the lower extremities. The fetus receives a mixture of oxygenated and deoxygenated blood.

This mixed blood reaches the fetal heart and begins the first of two bypass routes. Since the lungs do not oxygenate blood in the fetus they do not require the entire blood volume to pass through them. The first bypass route is through the **foramen ovale**, a hole between the right and left atria of the heart. Another bypass route occurs as the blood enters the **pulmonary trunk**. Blood moves from the pulmonary trunk through the **ductus arteriosus** and into the aortic arch.

Blood traveling back to the fetus is not fully deoxygenated but is a mixture of oxygenated and deoxygenated blood. This blood flows from the **internal iliac arteries** of the fetus and into the **umbilical arteries**. From the umbilical arteries the blood flows into the placenta.

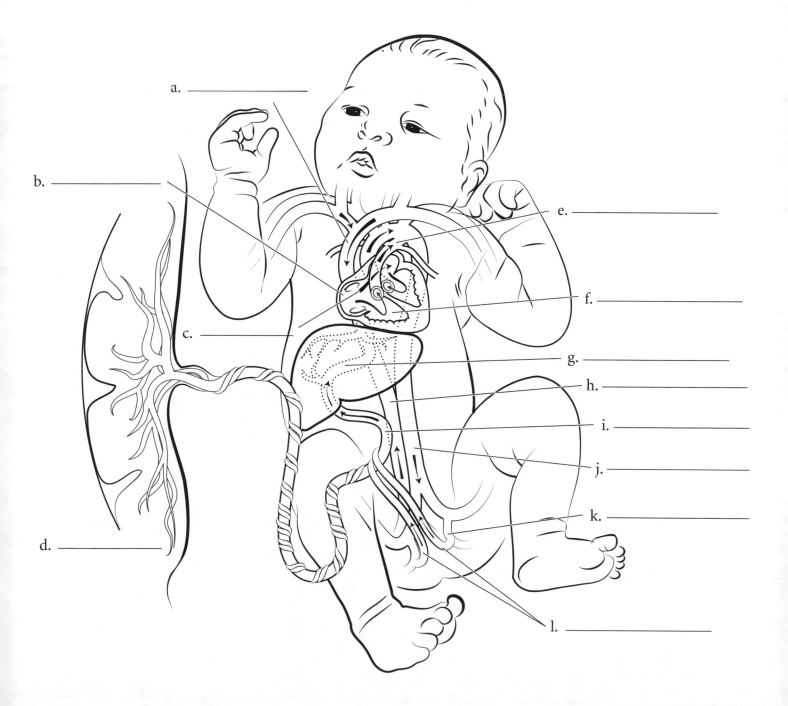

a. _____
b. _____
c. _____
d. _____
e. _____
f. _____
g. _____
h. _____
i. _____
j. _____
k. _____
l. _____

Answer Key: a. Superior vena cava, b. Right atrium, c. Foramen ovale, d. Placenta, e. Ductus arteriosus, f. Right ventricle, g. Ductus venosus, h. Inferior vena cava, i. Umbilical v., j. Abdominal aorta, k. Internal iliac a., l. Umbilical aa.

OVERVIEW OF THE LYMPH SYSTEM

The lymph system is composed of **lymphatics** or **lymph vessels** and glands and is a system with many functions. Fluid that bathes the cells (interstitial fluid) is returned to the cardiovascular system, in part, by the lymph system. This fluid, called **lymph**, passes through **lymph nodes** where impurities and foreign microbes are removed. Other parts of the lymph system include lymph organs such as the **spleen**. These organs produce cells that protect the body from foreign compounds, and have other immune functions such as cleansing the body of cellular debris and removing old blood cells from circulation.

The main exchange of fluid from the cardiovascular system occurs at the capillary level. **Arterioles** carry blood to the capillary bed and the **venules** return blood from the capillaries. About ninety percent of the fluid that flows from the blood capillaries to the interstices around the cells is reabsorbed by the capillaries. The remaining ten percent of the interstitial fluid enters the lymph system by **lymph capillaries** and travels through lymphatics. These lymph capillaries have one-way valves that allow the fluid to enter the lymphatics and not return to the cells. Once the fluid enters the lymphatic system it is called lymph. The lymph travels through the lymphatics and some of these merge into a large vessel in the abdomen called the **cisterna chyli**. This vessel, in turn, takes lymph to the **thoracic duct** that returns the lymph to the cardiovascular system. Label the structures of the lymph system and color them in.

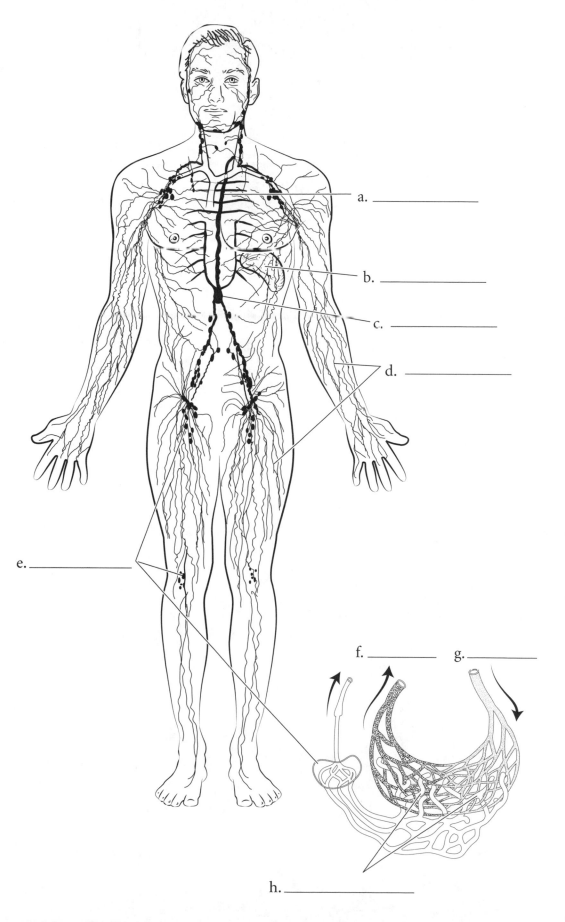

a. _____

b. _____

c. _____

d. _____

e. _____

f. _____   g. _____

h. _____

RETURN DRAINAGE

One of the functions of the lymph system is to return tissue fluid to the cardiovascular system.

The **right lymphatic duct** returns blood to the **right internal jugular vein**. This occurs at the junction where the **right subclavian vein** and the right internal jugular vein reach the right brachiocephalic vein. The **thoracic duct** enters the cardiovascular system at the point where the **left internal jugular vein** and the **left subclavian vein** enter the left brachiocephalic vein. **Lymph nodes** occur along the path and cleanse the lymph. The **thymus** is a lymph organ that occurs near these drainage areas. The thoracic duct receives lymph from most of the body while the right lymphatic duct receives lymph from the right side of the head, the right pectoral region, shoulder and right upper extremity. Label and color in the veins of the neck and upper thorax and label the lymphatic vessels that return fluid to the cardiovascular system.

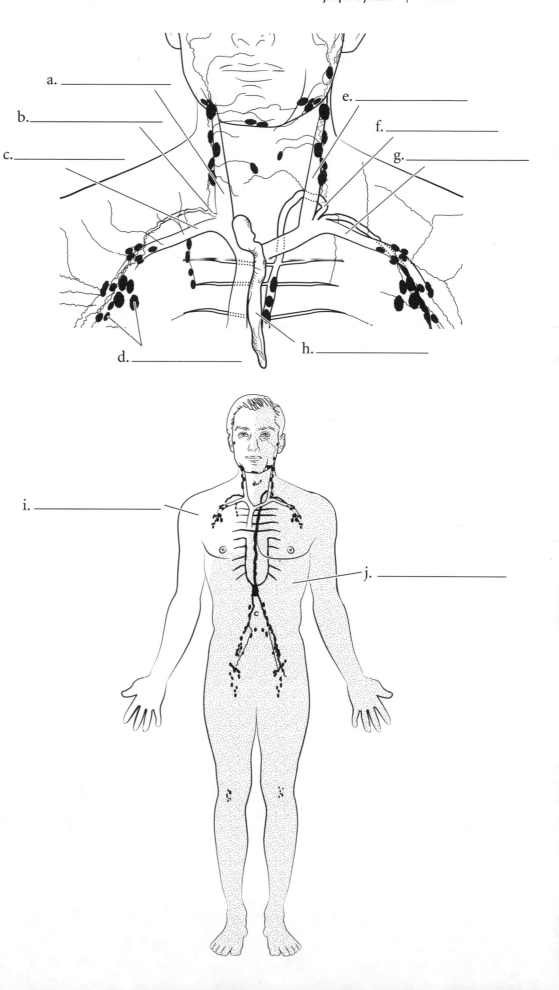

a. _____

b. _____

c. _____

d. _____

e. _____

f. _____

g. _____

h. _____

i. _____

j. _____

Answer Key: a. Right internal jugular vein, b. Right lymphatic duct, c. Right subclavian vein, d. Lymph nodes, e. Left internal jugular vein, f. Thoracic duct, g. Left subclavian vein, h. Thymus, i. Right drainage area, j. Left drainage area

TONSILS

The tonsils are lymph organs that provide protection against microbes entering the mouth and nose. Tonsils are regions of mucous membrane with lymph tissue. The **pharyngeal tonsils** are located in the naso-pharynx (a region posterior to the nasal cavity and superior to the oral cavity) and they provide some protection from inhaled material. The **lingual tonsils** are on the posterior part of the **tongue** and, along with the **palatine tonsils** on the side of the oral cavity, they provide protection from material that enters the body by mouth. These tonsils cluster to form a **tonsillar (Waldeyer's) ring** that protects the body from microbial invasion. Label the tonsils and associated structures and color them in.

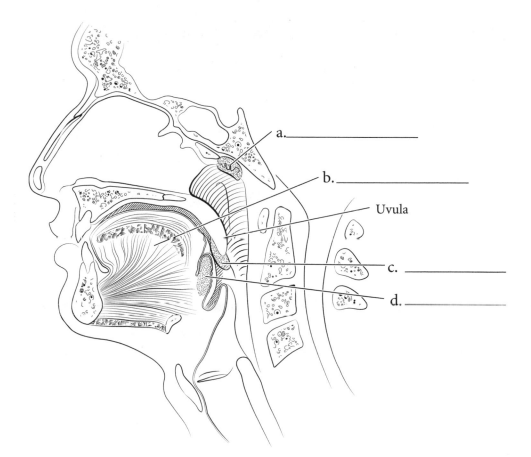

a._____

b._____

Uvula

c._____

d._____

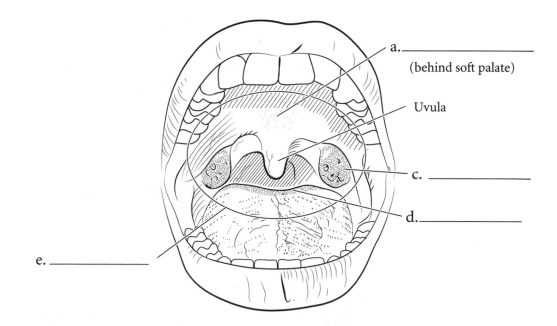

a._____
(behind soft palate)

Uvula

c._____

d._____

e._____

Answer Key: a. Pharyngeal tonsil, b. Tongue, c. Palatine tonsil, d. Lingual tonsil, e. Tonsillar (Waldeyer's) ring

SPLEEN

The **spleen** is on the left side of the body and is close to the pancreas. The **splenic artery** takes blood to the spleen and the **splenic vein** takes blood from the spleen. The spleen is important in removing aging red blood cells from circulation and recycling them. The spleen has both **red pulp** and **white pulp**. The red pulp is involved in red blood cell removal and the white pulp produces lymphocytes. The spleen has **splenic cords** that have lymphocytes along their length. Label the parts of the spleen and associated structures and color them in. Select red for the red pulp and leave the white pulp white.

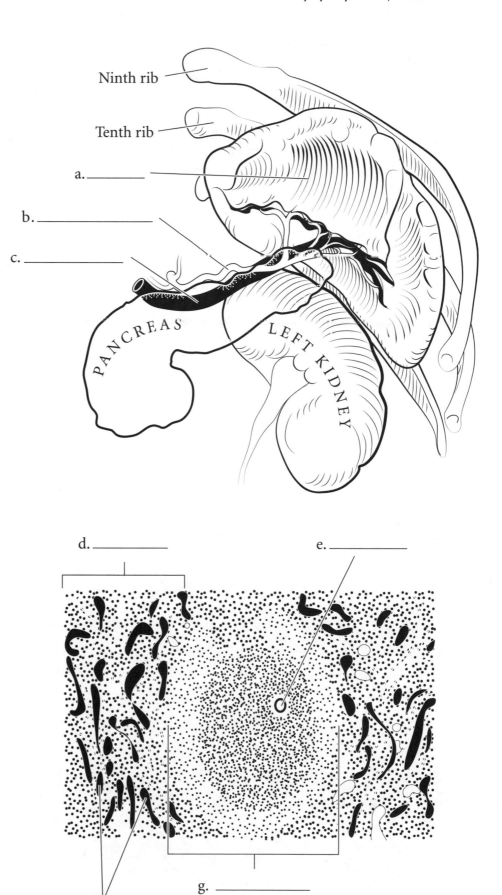

Ninth rib

Tenth rib

a. _____

b. _____

c. _____

PANCREAS

LEFT KIDNEY

d. _____

e. _____

f. _____

g. _____

(filled with red blood cells)

Answer Key: a. Spleen, b. Splenic artery, c. Splenic vein, d. Red pulp, e. Arteriole, f. Sinuses, g. White pulp

LYMPH NODES

Lymph nodes are found typically in clusters along the route that **lymphatics** take as lymph is returned to the cardiovascular system. **Afferent lymphatics** bring lymph to the node and **efferent lymphatics** receive lymph from the node.

Lymph nodes consist of an outer **cortex** and an inner **medulla**. The cortex produces lymphocytes and the medulla has **medullary cords** that have clusters of lymph cells that cleanse the lymph passing through the nodes. Label the lymphatics and parts of the lymph node and color them in.

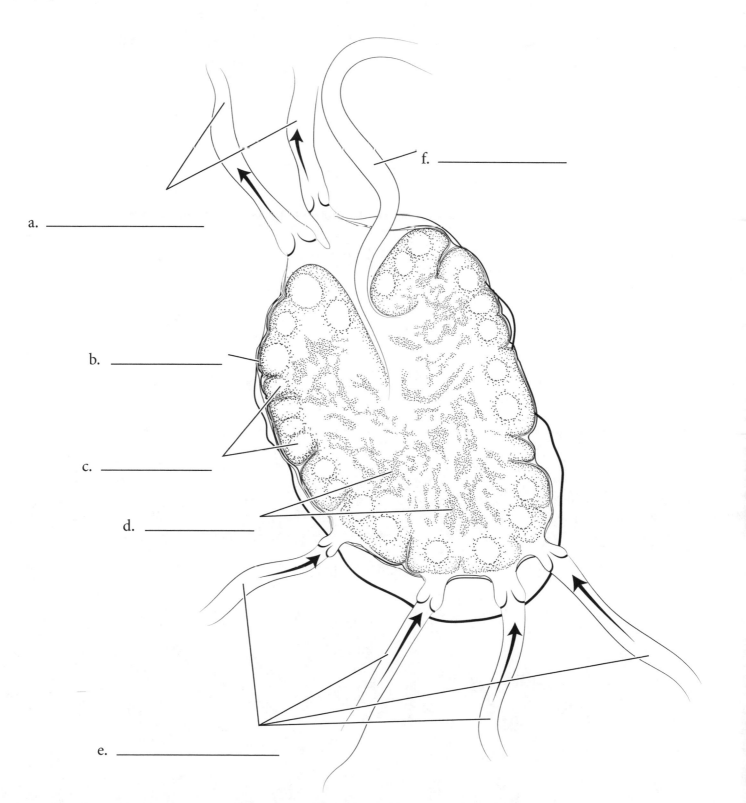

a. _____

f. _____

b. _____

c. _____

d. _____

e. _____

Answer Key: a. Efferent lymphatics, b. Capsule, c. Cortex, d. Medulla with medullary cords. e. Afferent lymphatics, f. Blood vessels

LACTEALS

The lymph system has a special function in digestion. Not only are there lymph nodes along parts of the digestive tract that protect the body from possible invasion from ingested microbes, but fatty acids from digestion are absorbed by special vessels called **lacteals**. Lacteals are found in the **small intestine** in finger-like structures called **villi**. These villi also contain **capillaries** which absorb sugars and amino acids. The lacteals absorb the fatty acids, products from the digestion of lipids in the diet. They travel through the **lymphatic vessels** to the cardiovascular system. Label the villi, capillaries, and lacteals and color them in.

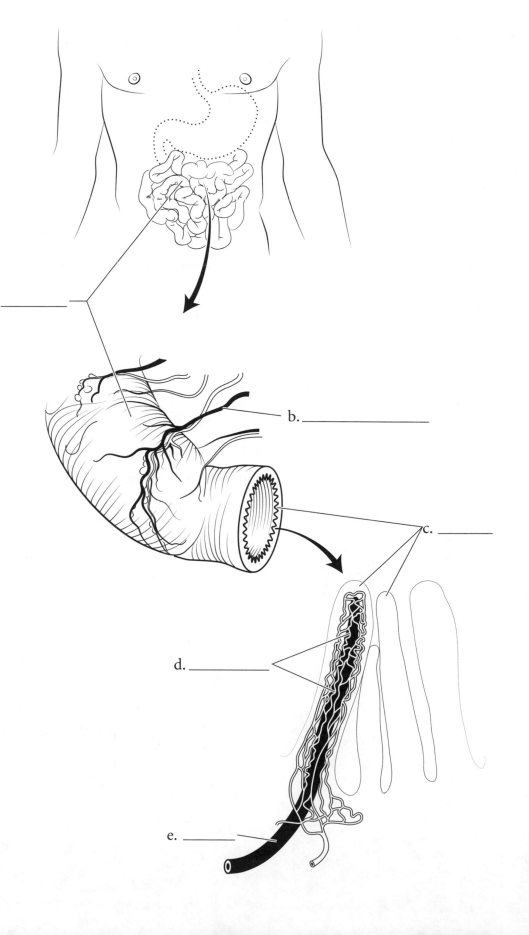

a. _____

b. _____

c. _____

d. _____

e. _____

Answer Key: a. Small intestine,
b. Lymphatic vessel, c. Villi,
d. Capillaries, e. Lacteal

TWO TYPES OF IMMUNITY

The body can control against foreign particles either by **cell-mediated immunity** or **antibody mediated immunity.** In antibody mediated immunity, foreign particles called **antigens** (typically proteins or carbohydrates on the surface of invading cells) stimulate **B cells** to become **plasma cells** and **memory B cells**. The plasma cells produce **antibodies** and these react with the antigens stimulating their destruction.

In cell-mediated immunity, the reacting cells are called **helper T cells** and they cause the activation of and the differentiation of other T cells into **memory T cells** and **effector** or **cytotoxic T cells**. The cytotoxic T cells can recognize foreign cells and destroy them. The steps in immune reactions are much more complex than this but this description provides a general understanding of the process. Fill in the illustration using the terms provided. Color the different cells and antibodies using one type of color (various types of orange for B cells) and another for T cells.

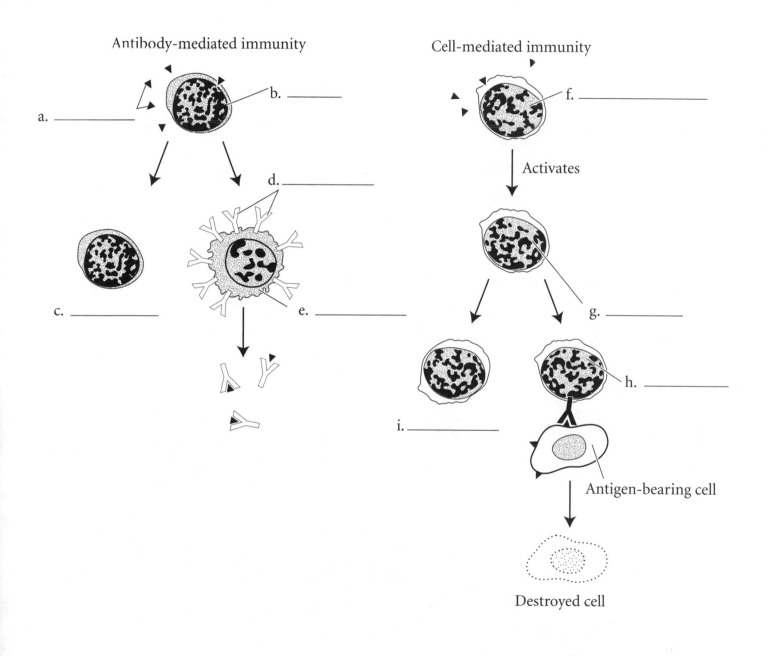

Antibody-mediated immunity

a. _____
b. _____
c. _____
d. _____
e. _____

Cell-mediated immunity

f. _____
Activates
g. _____
h. _____
i. _____

Antigen-bearing cell

Destroyed cell

Answer Key: a. Antigens, b. B cell, c. Memory B cell, d. Antibodies, e. Plasma cell, f. Helper T cell, g. Activated T cell, h. Effector (Cytotoxic) T cell, i. Memory T cell

OVERVIEW OF THE RESPIRATORY SYSTEM

The respiratory system consists of the **nose**, **nasal cavity**, **pharynx**, **larynx**, **trachea**, **lungs**, the linings of the lungs (**pleura**) and the respiratory muscles, such as the **diaphragm** and intercostal muscles. Label the respiratory figure and color in the major parts of the system.

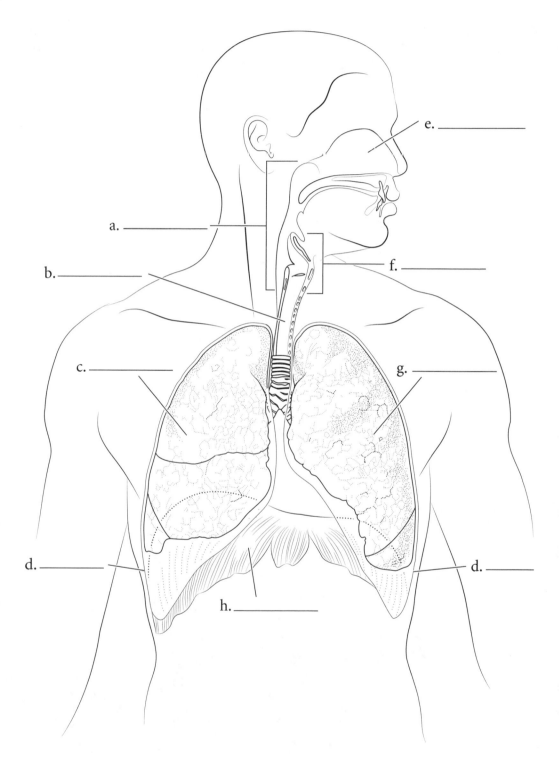

a. _____

b. _____

c. _____

d. _____

e. _____

f. _____

g. _____

d. _____

h. _____

Answer Key: a. Pharynx, b. Trachea, c. Right lung, d. Pleura, e. Nasal cavity, f. Larynx, g. Left lung, h. Diaphragm

LARYNX, TRACHEA, AND LUNGS OVERVIEW

Two main cartilages of the larynx can be seen from an anterior view. The **thyroid cartilage** is superior to the **cricoid cartilage**. Below the larynx is the **trachea** which divides into the **right** and **left primary bronchi**. The right primary bronchus leads to the **right lung** and the left primary

bronchus leads to the **left lung**. Label the parts of the respiratory system illustrated. Color the two visible cartilages of the larynx different colors and the trachea another color. Color the bronchi in first with a darker color and then color the lungs in with a lighter color.

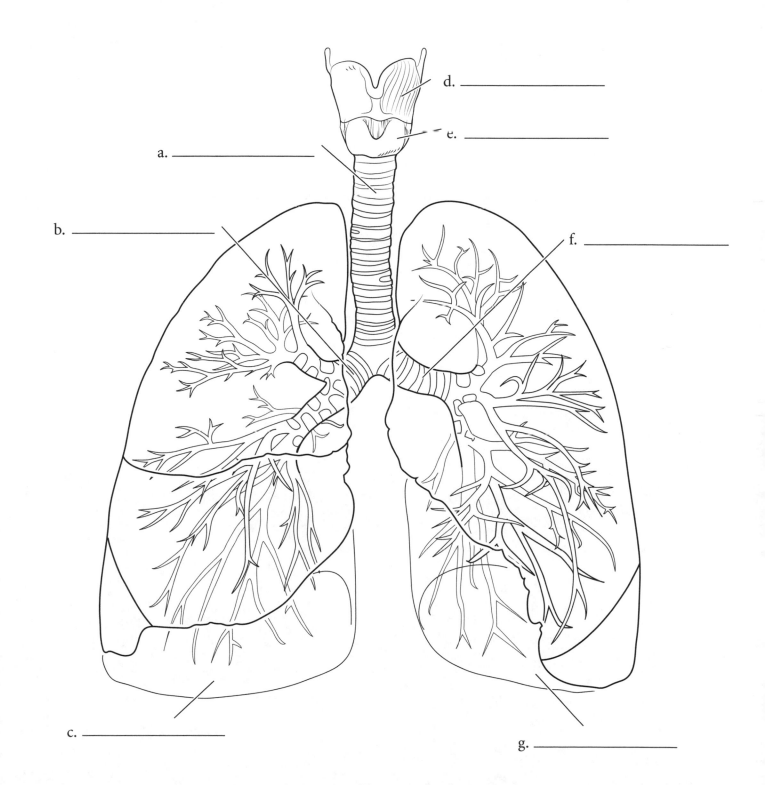

d. _____

e. _____

a. _____

b. _____

f. _____

c. _____

g. _____

Answer Key: a. Trachea, b. Right primary bronchus, c. Right lung, d. Thyroid cartilage, e. Cricoid cartilage, f. Left primary bronchus, g. Left lung

NOSE AND NASAL SEPTUM

The nose consists of the **nasal bones**, the **frontal process of the maxilla** at the root of the nose, and a number of cartilages. These nasal cartilages are made of hyaline cartilage. These are the **lateral nasal cartilages**, the **greater alar cartilages**, and the **lesser alar cartilages**. The **septal cartilage** also forms part of these cartilages. The openings of the nose (nostrils) are the **external nares** (**external naris** singular).

a. _____
b. _____
c. _____
d. _____
e. _____
f. _____
g. _____

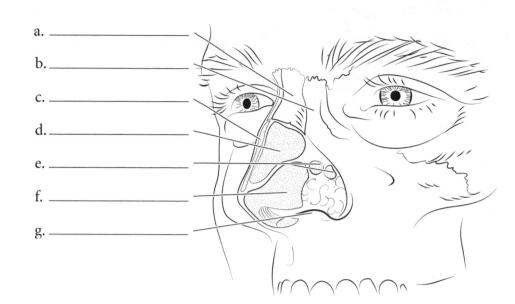

The nasal cavity has a wall that runs down the middle of it called the **nasal septum**. The septum consists of three parts, the **perpendicular plate of the ethmoid bone** (a continuation of the **crista galli**), the **vomer** and the **septal cartilage**. At the end of the nasal septum are two holes that separate the nasal cavity from the **nasopharynx**. These are the **choanae** or **internal nares**. The floor of the nasal cavity is bordered by the **hard palate** and the **soft palate**. At the junction of the crista galli and the perpendicular plate of the ethmoid is the **cribriform plate** of the ethmoid. Label the various structures of the nose such as the bones and color in the cartilages of the nose.

h. _____
i. _____
a. _____
j. _____
k. _____
c. _____
f. _____
l. _____
m. _____
n. _____

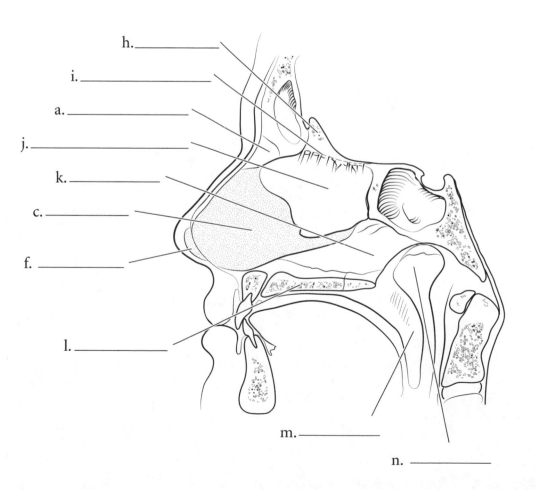

Answer Key: a. Nasal bone, b. Frontal process of maxilla, c. Septal cartilage, d. Lateral nasal cartilage, e. Lesser alar cartilages, f. Greater alar cartilage, g. External naris, h. Crista galli of ethmoid bone, i. Cribriform plate, j. Perpendicular plate of ethmoid bone, k. Vomer, l. Hard palate, m. Soft palate, n. Choanae (internal nares)

LATERAL WALL OF NASAL CAVITY AND RESPIRATORY EPITHELIUM

When looking at the nasal cavity, if the septal cartilage is removed you can see the **nasal conchae.** These structures force the inhaled air to come into contact with the wall of the nasal cavity where the air is warmed and moistened. There are three nasal conchae, the **superior nasal concha,** the **middle nasal concha,** and the **inferior nasal concha.** Note the position of the conchae with the **nasal bone,** the **hard palate** and the **soft palate.** Label the nasal cavity and the structures that are associated with the cavity.

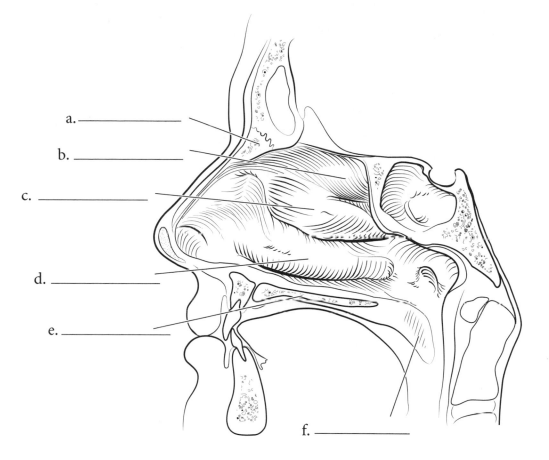

a. _____
b. _____
c. _____
d. _____
e. _____
f. _____

The nasal cavity is lined with **respiratory epithelium** which is **pseudostratified ciliated columnar epithelium** with **goblet cells.** Respiratory epithelium is found in the nasal cavity, the lower larynx, trachea, and bronchi. The goblet cells secrete **mucus** which forms a film over the epithelial surface. Dust and other particulate matter sticks to the **mucous sheet** which is moved by the **cilia.** This provides a protective function, removing particulate matter from entering the lungs where it might do damage. Label the various parts of respiratory epithelium such as the **nucleus, cilia, mucous sheet, goblet cells,** and **basement membrane.**

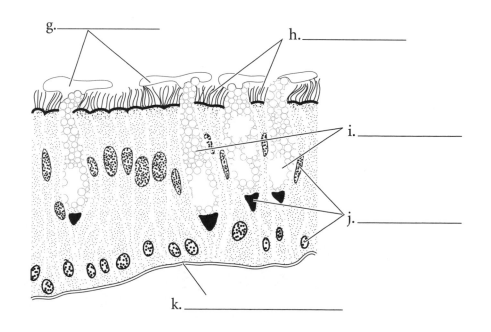

g. _____
h. _____
i. _____
j. _____
k. _____

Answer Key: a. Nasal bone, b. Superior nasal concha, c. Middle nasal concha, d. Inferior nasal concha, e. Hard palate, f. Soft palate, g. Mucous sheet, h. Cilia, i. Goblet cells, j. Nuclei, k. Basement membrane

CORONAL VIEW OF THE NASAL CONCHAE AND LARYNX

The nasal cavity is more than a hole behind the nose. Inhaled air swirls around the conchae and is warmed and moistened in the process. Label and color the **septal cartilage** in a coronal section of the nose. Label and color each of the conchae. The **superior nasal concha, middle nasal** concha, and the **inferior nasal concha** should each have a different color. The **frontal** and **ethmoid sinuses** can also be seen in this illustration. They give resonance to the voice. Note the location of the **hard palate** and the **external naris** in this coronal section. The larynx is also sectioned in this plane and the position of the **thyroid cartilage**, the **vocal fold**, the **cricoid cartilage**, and the **trachea** are seen in this view. Label and color the rest of the structures in this illustration.

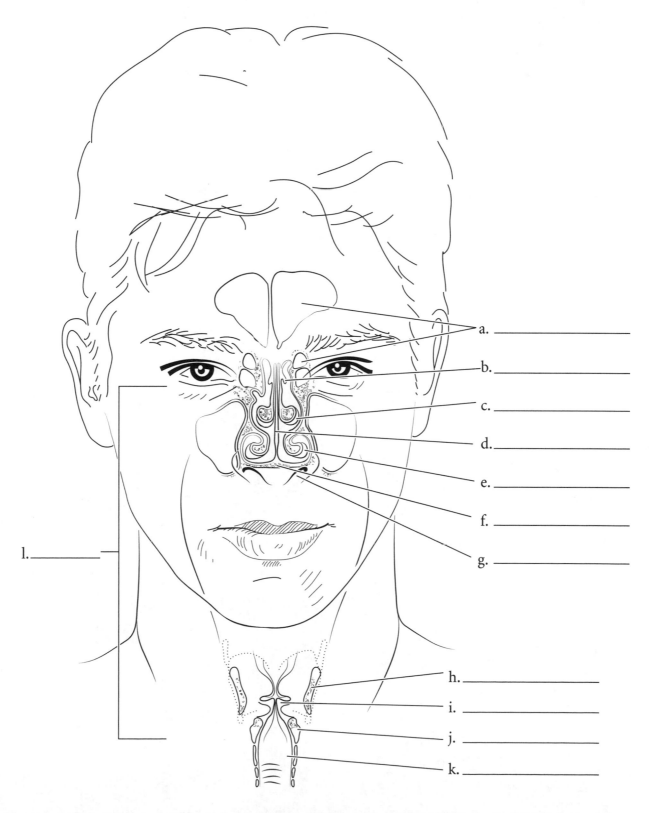

a. _____
b. _____
c. _____
d. _____
e. _____
f. _____
g. _____
h. _____
i. _____
j. _____
k. _____
l. _____

Answer Key: a. Sinuses, b. Superior nasal concha, c. Middle nasal concha, d. Septal cartilage, e. Inferior nasal concha, f. Hard palate, g. External naris, h. Thyroid cartilage, i. Vocal fold, j. Cricoid cartilage, k. Trachea

LARYNX AND TRACHEA

The **larynx** is the "voice box" and it not only produces sound for speech but also separates the flow of air to the lungs from the flow of foods and liquids that go down the esophagus. The **thyroid cartilage** is the largest cartilage of the larynx and it is easily seen from the anterior aspect. The thyroid cartilage is inferior to the **hyoid bone**. Behind the thyroid cartilage is the **epiglottis** which is the only laryngeal structure made of elastic cartilage. Inferior to the thyroid cartilage is the **cricoid cartilage** and it is the inferior border of the larynx. The **cricothyroid ligament** joins these anterior structures together. Above the cricoid cartilage are the paired **arytenoid cartilages**. These attach to the vocal folds and tighten them, causing the voice to increase in pitch. Superior to the arytenoid cartilages are the **corniculate cartilages** that are shaped like small horns. The **glottis** is the opening into the larynx and the **epiglottis** is the flap that folds over the glottis during swallowing.

In the midsagittal section of the larynx you can see that the **cricoid cartilage** is larger on the posterior aspect. The **thyroid cartilage** is prominent on the anterior side, the **arytenoid** and **corniculate cartilages** are prominent on the posterior side, along with the **cricoid cartilage**, the **epiglottis**, and the vocal folds. The **vestibular fold** (**false vocal cord**) is superior and is found on the lateral wall of the larynx. Below this is the **vocal cord** (**vocal fold**) that produces sound. The **conus elasticus** consists of elastic tissue and connects the vocal folds to the cartilages. Below the larynx is the **trachea** which leads from the larynx to the lungs. Label and color the structures of the larynx and label and color in the trachea.

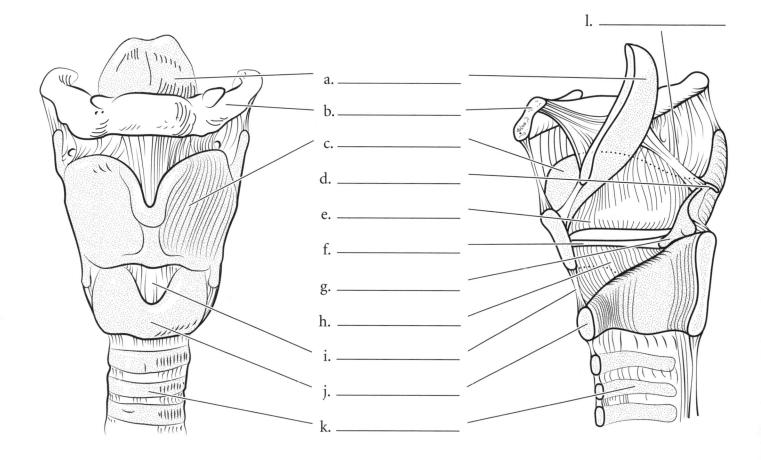

a. _____
b. _____
c. _____
d. _____
e. _____
f. _____
g. _____
h. _____
i. _____
j. _____
k. _____
l. _____

Answer Key: a. Epiglottis, b. Hyoid bone, c. Thyroid cartilage, d. Corniculate cartilage, e. Vestibular fold, f. Vocal fold, g. Arytenoid cartilage, h. Conus elasticus, i. Cricothyroid ligament, j. Cricoid cartilage, k. Trachea, l. Glottis

THE TRACHEA AND BRONCHIAL TREE

The **trachea** connects to the larynx superiorly and ends inferiorly in a keel-shaped structure called the **carina**. The trachea is composed of the **tracheal rings** which are hyaline cartilage. The posterior surface of the trachea has smooth muscle called the **trachealis muscle** that allows for the food in the esophagus to bulge into the trachea. The trachea branches into the **right primary bronchus** and the **left primary bronchus** which form part of the lungs.

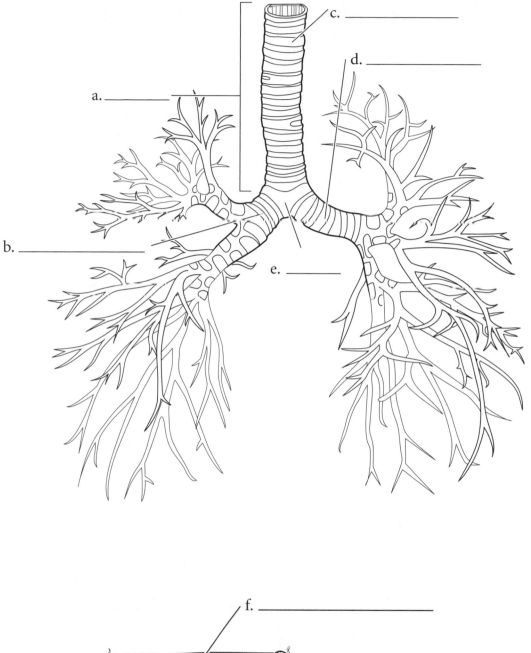

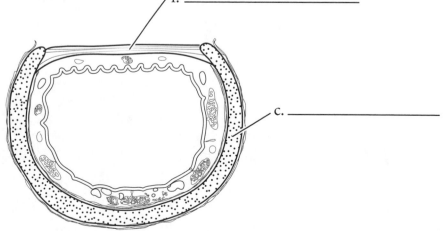

Answer Key: a. Trachea, b. Right primary bronchus, c. Tracheal ring, d. Left primary bronchus, e. Carina, f. Trachealis muscle

LUNGS AND MEMBRANES

The lungs are in the **thoracic cavity** on either side of the mediastinum. The membrane that occurs on the inside of the ribs and on the superior aspect of the diaphragm is known as the **parietal pleura**. The space inside of this is the **pleural cavity** and the lungs occupy the pleural cavities. The innermost membrane is the **visceral pleura** and it is attached to the surface of the lung. The right lung has three lobes: a **superior lobe**, a **middle lobe**, and an **inferior lobe**. The left lung has two lobes: a **superior lobe** and an **inferior lobe**. The left lung also has an indentation where the heart protrudes into the left lung and this is the **cardiac notch**. Label the membranes and the parts of the lungs and color them in.

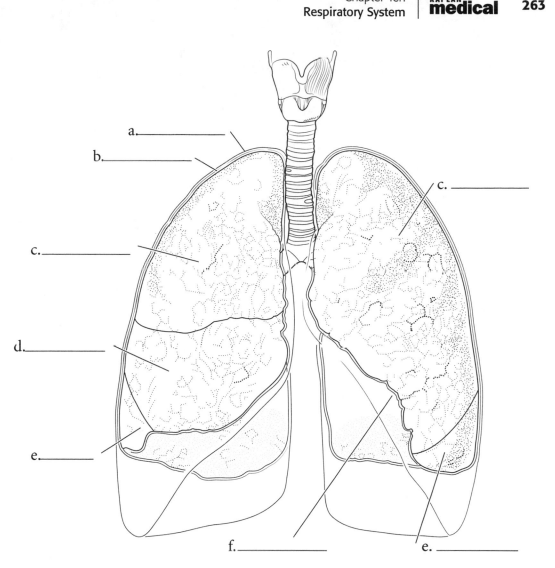

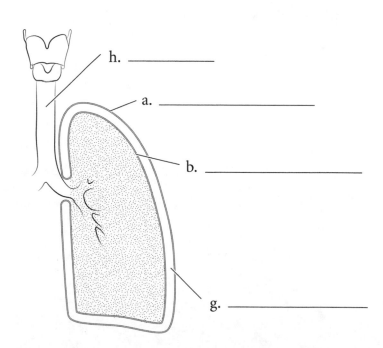

Answer Key: a. Parietal pleura,
b. Visceral pleura, c. Superior lobe,
d. Middle lobe, e. Inferior lobe,
f. Cardiac notch, g. Pleural cavity,
h. Trachea

THE PATHWAY OF AIR

The lungs are like large sponges filled with microscopic spaces. Air travels to these spaces by the **bronchial tree**. The trachea splits at the level of the lungs into two **primary bronchi**. Each lung has a primary bronchus that divides to **secondary bronchi**. These divide further to **tertiary bronchi** which divide into smaller branches. Finally bronchi become **bronchioles** and these lead to smaller sacs where the exchange of oxygen and carbon dioxide occurs between the lungs and blood. Shade the major segments of the bronchial tree.

The air from the bronchioles moves into the **alveolar ducts** which are part of the clusters called **alveolar sacs**. The air flows into the alveolar duct which is a conduit to the individual **alveoli** (**alveolus** singular) and these are the areas where there is an exchange of oxygen and carbon dioxide between the air and blood. **Capillaries** are situated next to the alveoli and there are two thin set of membranes—one of the alveolus and one of the capillary—that allow the exchange of oxygen and carbon dioxide. Additionally there are **type II alveolar cells** (**septal cells**) that secrete a material called **surfactant**. This substance reduces the surface tension of the lungs, allowing them to expand more easily. Color in the structures of the alveolar sacs and the associated structures.

a. _____
b. _____
c. _____
d. _____
e. _____
f. _____

g. _____
h. _____
k. _____
i. _____
j. _____
k. _____

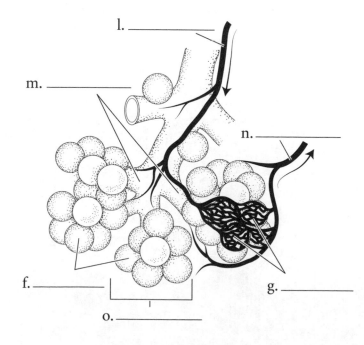

l. _____
m. _____
n. _____
f. _____
g. _____
o. _____

Answer Key: a. Cartilage, b. Secondary bronchus, c. Tertiary bronchus, d. Bronchi, e. Bronchioles, f. Alveoli, g. Capillaries, h. Type II alveolar cell (septal cell), i. Surfactant, j. Red blood cell, k. Alveolus, l. Pulmonary artery, m. Alveolar ducts, n. Pulmonary vein, o. Alveolar sac

OVERVIEW OF THE DIGESTIVE SYSTEM

The digestive system is composed of a long tube called the **alimentary canal** and the **accessory organs** including the liver, pancreas, and gall bladder. The alimentary canal starts at the mouth, includes the esophagus, stomach, intestines, and rectum and terminates at the **anus**. It can be defined as the tube through which ingested products move. The accessory organs have digestive functions but they do not come into contact with material passing through the digestive tract. The alimentary canal consists of numerous organs including the **mouth** which is the opening to the system and is directly anterior to the oral cavity. The terminal aspect of the oral cavity is defined by the small mass of fleshy tissue called the uvula. Posterior to the oral cavity is the oropharynx. This chamber receives food and liquid from the mouth and air from both the mouth and nasal cavity. The oropharynx leads to the **esophagus** which is a muscular tube that takes ingested material to the **stomach**. The stomach is a storage organ leading to the **small intestine** where material is digested and absorbed. The **large intestine** receives material from the small intestine, removes a significant amount of water, and stores the fecal material prior to defecation.

The **salivary glands** are the most superior accessory glands. They lubricate food and add digestive enzymes to material that is swallowed. The **liver**, **pancreas** and **gall bladder** all add secretions to the ingested material and aid in the digestive process. Label the parts of the digestive system, including the alimentary canal and the accessory organs, and color the individual digestive organs a different color.

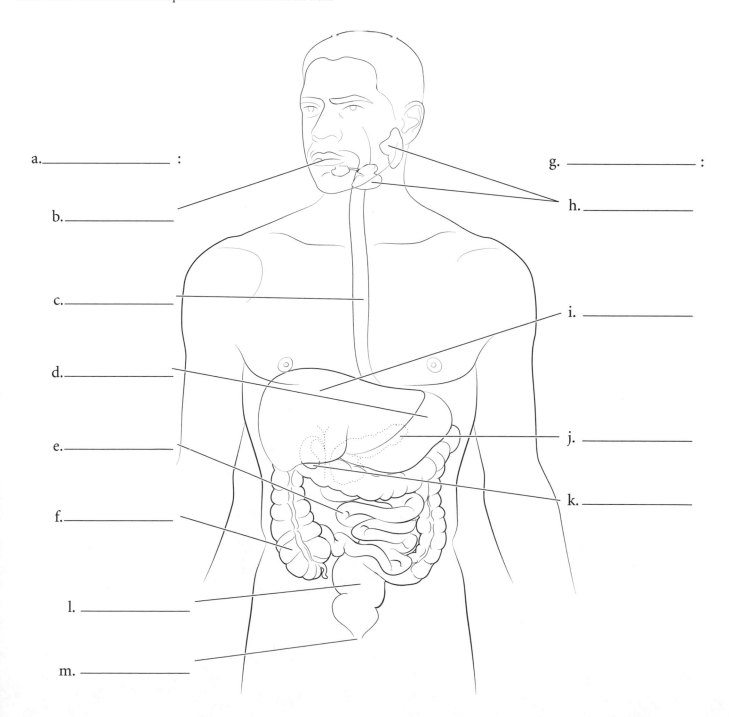

a._____ :

b._____

c._____

d._____

e._____

f._____

l. _____

m. _____

g. _____ :

h. _____

i. _____

j. _____

k. _____

Answer Key: a. Alimentary canal, b. Mouth, c. Esophagus, d. Stomach, e. Small intestine, f. Large intestine, g. Accessory organs, h. Salivary glands, i. Liver, j. Pancreas, k. Gall bladder, l. Rectum, m. Anus

MOUTH AND ORAL CAVITY

The mouth is the entrance to the digestive system. It is bordered by the two **labia** or lips. Each labium has a **labial frenulum** (**superior** and **inferior**) that holds the lip to the **gingiva**. The gingiva (gums) have a surface tissue of stratified squamous epithelium which is the cell type that lines the entire oral cavity. The oral cavity encloses the teeth, and the **tongue.** It is bordered by the **hard palate**, the **soft palate**, the **uvula**, the cheek walls, the muscles and associated tissue that spans across the bodies of the mandible. The oral cavity leads to the **oropharynx**, which in turn leads to the **esophagus**.

The **tongue** is a large muscle in the oral cavity that pushes food to the posterior part of the oral cavity for swallowing and helps form speech. It is held to the floor of the oral cavity by the lingual frenulum.

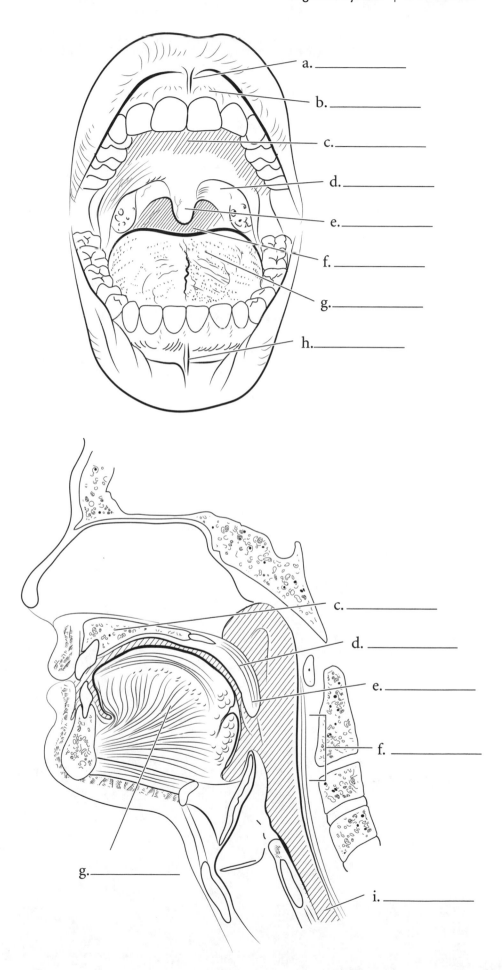

a. _____
b. _____
c. _____
d. _____
e. _____
f. _____
g. _____
h. _____

c. _____
d. _____
e. _____
f. _____
g. _____
i. _____

Answer Key: a. Superior labial frenulum, b. Gingiva, c. Hard palate, d. Soft palate, e. Uvula, f. Oropharynx, g. Tongue , h. Inferior labial frenulum, i. Esophagus

SALIVARY GLANDS

The three pair of salivary glands secrete saliva inside the oral cavity. The largest pair consists of the **parotid glands** and they are located just anterior to the ears. The **parotid duct** leads from the gland to posterior to the upper second molar. The **submandibular glands** are located inferior to the mandible and they take secretions to either side of the lingual frenulum. The **sublingual glands** are inferior to the tongue and have many tubes that lead to the lower oral cavity. Label the salivary glands and the parotid duct. Color each gland a different color.

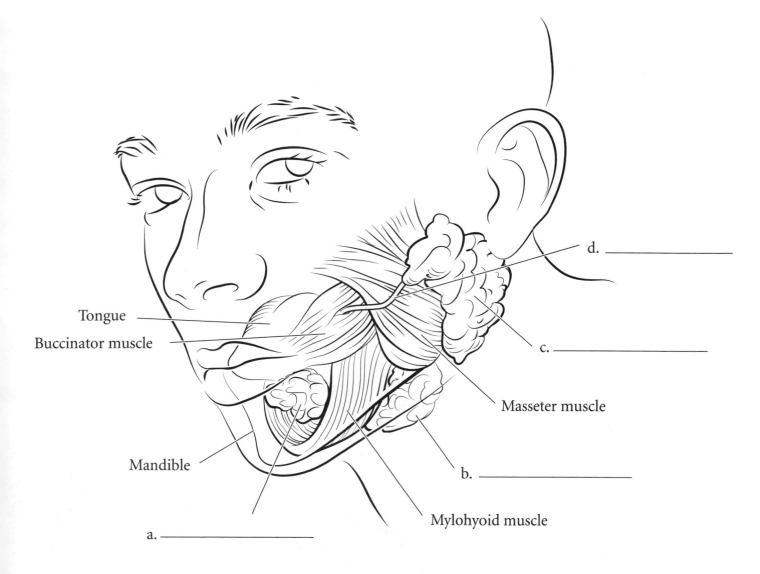

Tongue

Buccinator muscle

Mandible

a. _____

d. _____

c. _____

Masseter muscle

b. _____

Mylohyoid muscle

Answer Key: a. Sublingual gland, b. Submandibular gland, c. Parotid gland, d. Parotid duct

TEETH

The tooth has three general regions: the crown, the neck, and the root. The **crown** is the part of the tooth that erupts from the gums into the oral cavity. The **neck** is normally at the level of the gingiva and the **root** is imbedded into the bone. The tooth fits into the alveolar socket of the maxilla or the mandible and is held there by the **periodontal ligaments**.

The internal anatomy of the tooth reveals the hard **enamel** which is an extremely dense material that resists wear and abrasion. Deep to this is the **dentin**, a material similar to bone that provides the major structure of the tooth. In the root, the dentin is coated with **cementum** that helps fix the tooth in the alveolar socket. Inside of the dentin is the **pulp cavity** that houses **nerves** and **blood vessels**. These structures enter the tooth by the **apical foramen** and make their way to the pulp cavity by the **root canal**.

Humans have two series of teeth. Early in development come the **deciduous (milk) teeth**. The **permanent teeth** emerge as the skull is increasing in size. In deciduous teeth there are **incisors**, **cuspids (canines)**, and **molar teeth** but there are no premolars. In adults there are the **incisor teeth**, the **cuspids**, **premolars (bicuspids)**, and **molar teeth**. Label the parts of the tooth and then color in the regions of the tooth on one side of the illustration and the enamel, dentin, and other features on the other part of the illustration. For the deciduous and permanent teeth, use the same color for the incisors on both illustrations. Use another color for the cuspids and another for the premolars, and so on for the rest of the teeth.

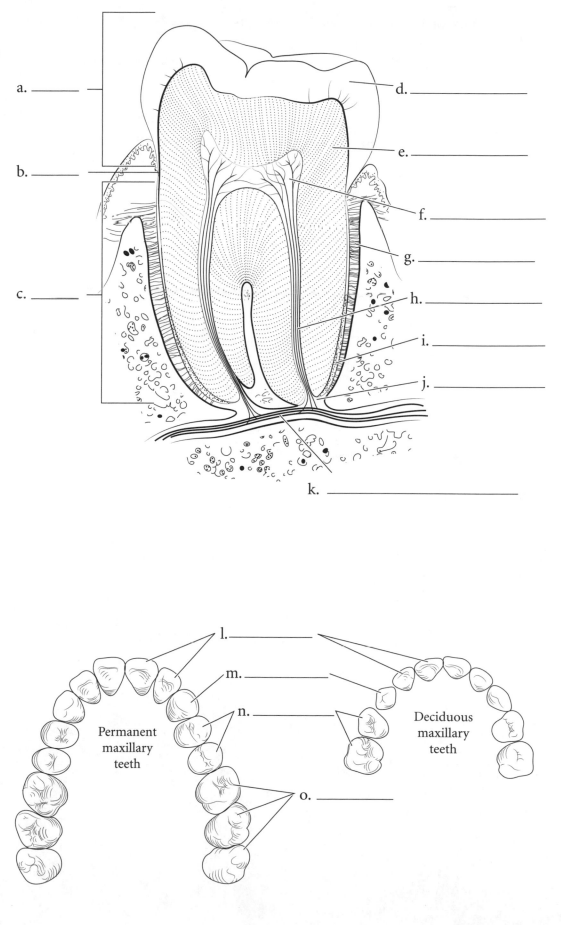

a. _____

b. _____

c. _____

d. _____

e. _____

f. _____

g. _____

h. _____

i. _____

j. _____

k. _____

l. _____

m. _____

n. _____

o. _____

Permanent maxillary teeth

Deciduous maxillary teeth

Answer Key: a. Crown, b. Neck, c. Root, d. Enamel, e. Dentin, f. Pulp cavity, g. Periodontal ligament, h. Root canal, i. Cementum, j. Apical foramen, k. Blood vessels and nerves, l. Incisors, m. Cuspids (canines), n. Premolars (bicuspids), o. Molars

ESOPHAGUS

Food moves from the **oral cavity** to the **oropharynx** by action of the tongue. The **uvula** flips upward keeping the food from entering the nasal cavity. Food passes from the oropharynx into the laryngopharynx before moving to the esophagus. The food enters the **esophagus** as a lump or **bolus** and passes through the **esophageal sphincter** to the stomach. Once it enters the stomach the bolus mixes with stomach fluid and becomes a liquid called chyme. Label and color the structures leading to the esophagus and the esophagus itself including the esophageal sphincter.

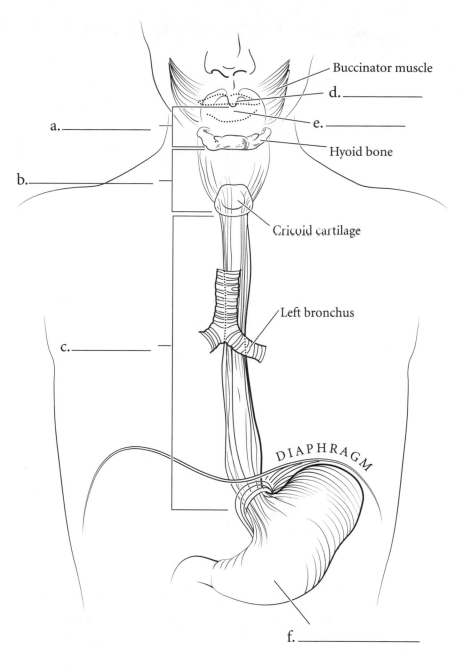

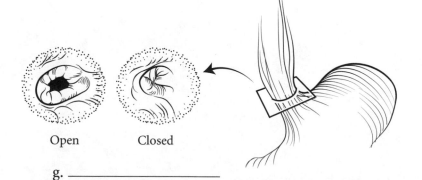

Open   Closed

STOMACH

The stomach is located on the left side of the body, just inferior to the diaphragm. It is the part of the alimentary canal located between the esophagus and the small intestine. The stomach has an upper **cardia** and a small domed portion called the **fundus**. The stomach contents are restricted from flowing back into the esophagus by the esophageal sphincter. If stomach fluid refluxes into the esophagus, it is felt as "heartburn."

The main portion of the stomach is the **body** and the narrow region, leading to the **duodenum** is the **antrum** or **pyloric region**. This leads to the **pyloric canal** which is controlled by the **pyloric sphincter**. The **greater curvature** is located on the left edge of the stomach and the **lesser curvature** is on the right side. The stomach has inner ridges called **rugae** which allow for expansion of the stomach.

The stomach has many layers. The inner layer is called the **mucosa** which is rich in glands that secrete acids and inactive enzymes such as pepsinogen into the stomach cavity. Pepsinogen is activated by hydrochloric acid. The mucosa has **gastric pits** with **parietal cells** and **chief cells** emptying into the pits. The parietal cells secrete hydrochloric acid and the chief cells secrete pepsinogen. External to the mucosa is the **submucosa** and this layer has many blood vessels imbedded in connective tissue. Beyond this is the **muscularis**. In the stomach there are three layers of the muscularis. These are the **oblique layer**, **circular layer**, and **longitudinal layer**. The most external layer is the **serosa** (also known as the **visceral peritoneum**) and this is next to the abdominal cavity. Label the parts of the stomach and color them in. Color the layers of the muscularis using different colors of red or pink for each layer. Color the general regions of the stomach different colors along with the separate sphincters.

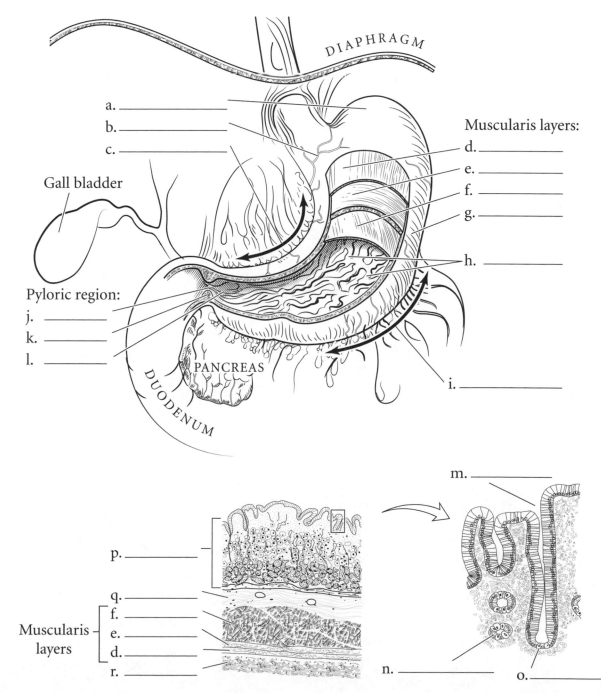

Answer Key: a. Fundus, b. Cardia, c. Lesser curvature, d. Longitudinal layer (of muscularis), e. Circular layer (of muscularis), f. Oblique layer (of muscularis), g. Body, h. Rugae, i. Greater curvature, j. Pyloric canal, k. Pyloric sphincter, l. Antrum, m. Gastric pit, n. Chief cell, o. Parietal cell, p. Mucosa, q. Submucosa, r. Serosa

SMALL INTESTINE

The small intestine receives the contents of the stomach, continues the process of digestion and absorbs nutrients. The first part of the small intestine is the **duodenum**, a short tube of about twelve inches in length, that receives material from the stomach, enzymes and buffers from the **pancreas**, and bile from the **gall bladder**. The duodenum has **circular folds** in the wall that increase the surface area. The **jejunum** is the next section of the small intestine and it makes up about forty percent of the small intestine. There are **circular folds** in the jejunum as well. The **ileum** is the terminal portion of the small intestine and represents about sixty percent of the small intestine. The small intestine is small in diameter and that is how it gets its name.

The small intestine is distinguished from the rest of the alimentary canal by the presence of **villi**. These small structures in the mucosa increase the surface area of the small intestine and house blood capillaries and lacteals for the absorption of nutrients. The small intestine has the four layers typical of the other organs of the gastrointestinal tract: the mucosa, **submucosa**, **muscularis**, and serosa. Label the parts of the small intestine and color in the various regions and layers of the small intestine.

a. _____   b. _____

c. _____

STOMACH

c. _____

d. _____
(Upper two-fifths)

CECUM

e. _____
(Lower three-fifths)

f. _____

g. _____

h. _____

i. _____

d. _____   e. _____

Answer Key: a. Gall bladder, b. Pancreas, c. Duodenum, d. Jejunum, e. Ileum, f. Circular fold, g. Villi, h. Submucosa, i. Muscularis

LARGE INTESTINE

The large intestine is shorter than the small intestine but has greater width. The large intestine begins in the lower right quadrant of the abdomen with a sac-like structure called the **cecum**. The ileocecal valve is a muscular sphincter that prevents the fecal material in the cecum from flowing back into the ileum. At this junction is the **vermiform appendix**. Material in the large intestine moves from the cecum to the **ascending colon** and then makes a sharp turn at the **hepatic flexure**. Once this turn is accomplished, the material is in the **transverse colon**. From here there is a sharp downward angle called the **splenic flexure** and the material enters the **descending colon**. From the descending colon, the material enters an S-shaped tube called the **sigmoid colon** and then enters the **rectum**. The rectum is the end of the large intestine. The rectum leads to the **anal canal** which is a short tube leading to the **anus**.

There are several anatomical features that separate the large intestine from the small intestine. The large intestine has long strips of smooth muscle that run the length of the large intestine. These are called the **teniae coli**. These muscles pull the intestine into small compartments called **haustra**. Another distinguishing feature of the large intestine is the presence of small fat globules called **epiploic appendages**. Label the parts of the large intestine and color in each region with a different color. Color the haustra light red and the tenia coli pink. Color the epiploic appendages yellow.

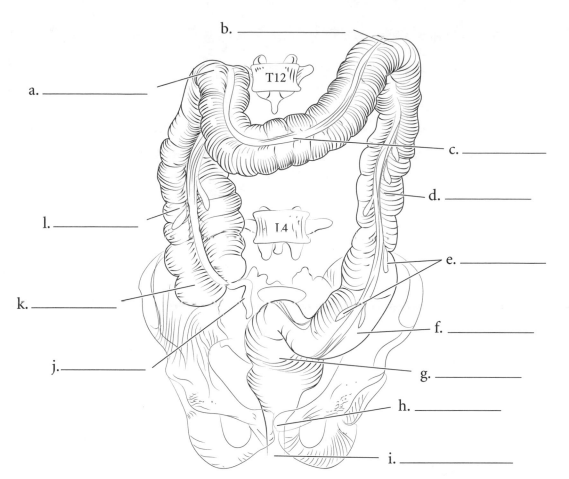

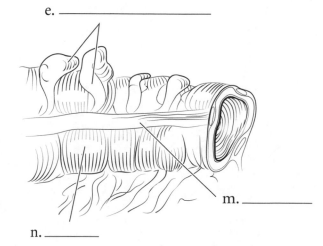

LIVER

The liver is the largest internal organ of the body. It is on the right side of the body and plays a major metabolic function in digestion and also in processing material from the blood. The liver has four lobes in humans and is held to the diaphragm by the **falciform ligament**. The **right lobe** is the largest of the lobes. The **left lobe** is also reasonably large. The **quadrate lobe** is anterior and is rectangular in shape when seen from the inferior view. The **caudate lobe** is a posterior lobe of the liver.

The blood flows into the liver from two sources. The **hepatic portal vein** takes blood to the liver from the digestive tract and some abdominal organs. The **hepatic artery** brings oxygenated blood to the liver. The liver is composed of microscopic sections called **liver lobules**. These are typically hexagonal columns that have a **central vein** that takes blood back to the heart via the hepatic vein. Blood travels to the central vein by **sinusoids**, canals that are lined by **hepatocytes** (liver cells). Hepatocytes clean the blood or process material in the blood. Old blood pigments are recycled by the liver and are converted to bile. The bile moves through **bile canaliculi** and eventually is stored in the gall bladder. The branches of the hepatic artery, portal vein, and **bile duct** are clustered together and form the **portal triad**. Label the liver structures on the illustrations. Color in the lobes of the liver using different colors for each lobe. Color the hepatic portal vein blue, the hepatic artery red, and the bile ducts green.

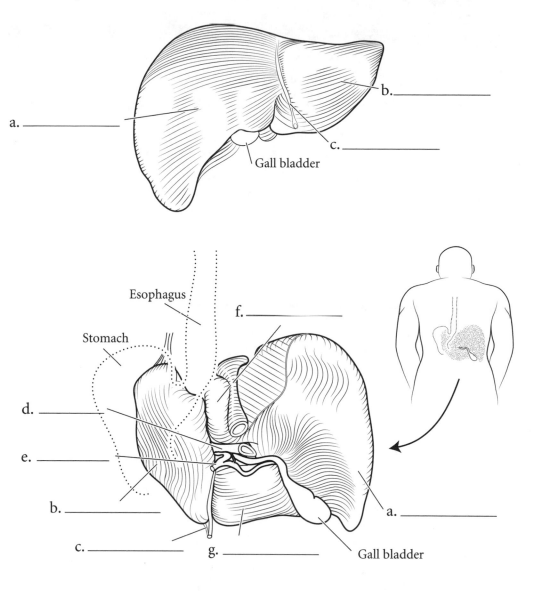

Liver Lobule

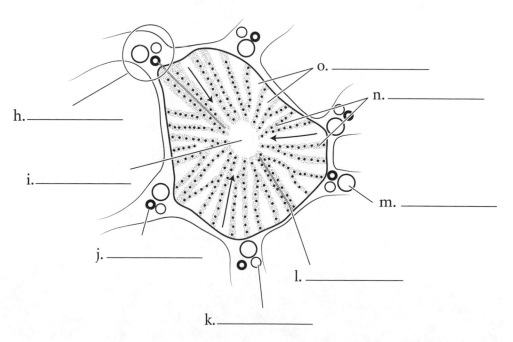

Answer Key: a. Right lobe, b. Left lobe, c. Falciform ligament, d. Portal vein, e. Hepatic artery, f. Caudate lobe, g. Quadrate lobe, h. Portal triad, i. Central vein, j. Bile duct, k. Hepatic artery branch, l. Bile canaliculus, m. Portal vein branch, n. Hepatocytes, o. Sinusoids

PANCREAS/ GALL BLADDER

The **pancreas** is a complex organ that has both a digestive function and an endocrine function. The digestive function of the pancreas consists of producing enzymes for the digestion of materials in the small intestine and the secretion of buffers to increase the pH of the fluid secreted from the stomach. The pancreas has a **head**, next to the duodenum, a main **body** and a **tail** near the spleen. The enzymes and buffers secreted into the small intestine flow into the **pancreatic duct** before entering the small intestine.

The **gall bladder** receives bile from the **liver**, storing and condensing it prior to secreting it into the small intestine. Bile is an emulsifier of fats, making them disperse in the liquid chyme of the digestive tract. Bile flows from the **left** and **right hepatic ducts**, into the **common hepatic duct**, into the **cystic duct** then entering the gall bladder. When the gall bladder contracts, bile moves back out the cystic duct and into the **common bile duct** before entering the small intestine. Usually the common bile duct and the pancreatic duct join before they enter the small intestine. In this case the tube is called the **hepatopancreatic ampulla** and it leads to the **duodenal papilla**. Label the parts of the pancreas, gall bladder and ducts and color them in.

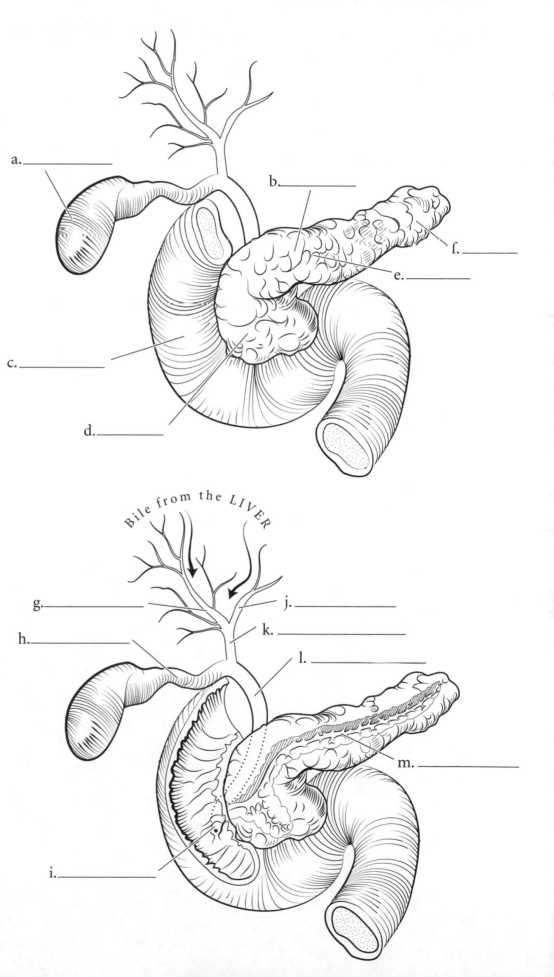

Bile from the LIVER

Answer Key: a. Gall bladder, b. Pancreas, c. Duodenum, d. Head, e. Body, f. Tail, g. Right hepatic duct, h. Cystic duct, i. Duodenal papilla, j. Left hepatic duct, k. Common hepatic duct, l. Common bile duct, m. Pancreatic duct

OVERVIEW OF THE URINARY SYSTEM

The urinary system consists of two **kidneys**, two **ureters**, a **urinary bladder**, and a **urethra**. The right kidney is a little more inferior than the left kidney due to the presence of the liver on the right side of the body. The kidneys are located near the twelfth vertebra and extend to the third lumbar vertebra. They receive blood from the **renal artery**. The kidneys are retroperitoneal, meaning that they are posterior to the parietal peritoneum. The ureters are also retroperitoneal and take urine to the bladder. Since the urinary bladder is located anterior to the parietal peritoneum it is called anteperitoneal. Label the organs of the urinary system and use separate colors for the kidneys, ureters, urinary bladder, and urethra.

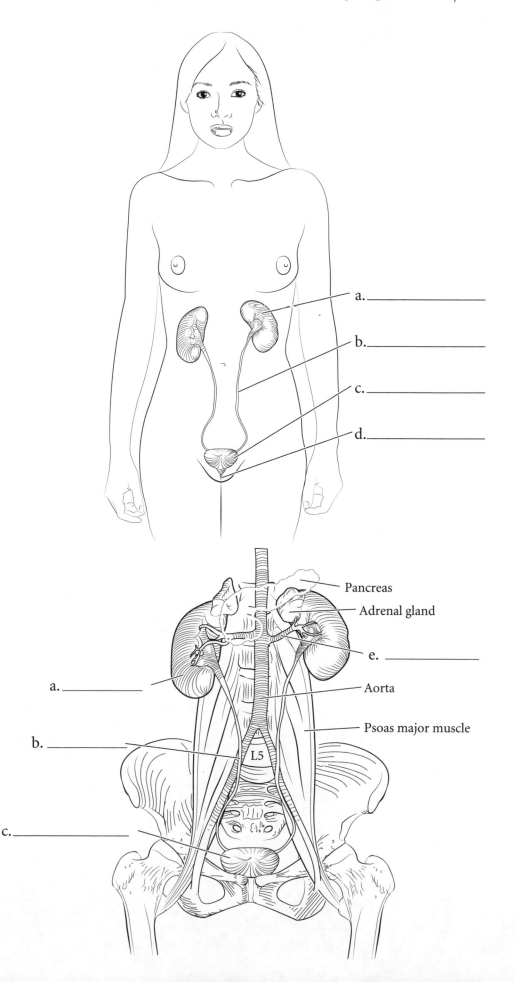

a. _____

b. _____

c. _____

d. _____

Pancreas

Adrenal gland

e. _____

Aorta

Psoas major muscle

a. _____

b. _____

L5

c. _____

Answer Key: a. Kidney, b. Ureter,
c. Urinary bladder, d. Urethra,
e. Renal artery

KIDNEY

The kidney is a bean-shaped organ. The outer surface of the kidney is covered by the **renal capsule**. The depression on the medial side is the **hilum** where the **renal artery** enters the kidney and the **renal vein** and the **ureter** exit. The kidney is sectioned in the coronal plane to study the internal anatomy. The renal capsule is a thin membrane on the exterior of the kidney. Deep to the capsule is the **renal cortex** where filtration takes place in the kidney. The **renal medulla** is deep to the cortex and it is divided into **renal columns** and **renal pyramids**. Each pyramid ends in a **papilla** and this drips urine into small funnel-shaped structures called the **minor calyces** (*calyx* singular). The minor calyces join to form the **major calyces** and these, in turn, take urine to the **renal pelvis**. The renal pelvis occupies most of the **renal sinus**, a space in the kidney. The renal pelvis takes urine to the ureter on the medial side of the kidney. Blood travels to the kidney by the **renal artery**. From there the blood moves into **segmental arteries** and then **interlobar arteries**. From the interlobar arteries the blood travels to the **arcuate arteries**. These arteries are the dividing structures between the renal cortex and the renal medulla. From the arcuate arteries blood flows into the **interlobular arteries**. Label the parts of the kidney and associated structures. Use one color for the cortex and different shades of another color for the renal pyramids and columns. Color the renal artery red and the renal vein blue. Use yellow for the pelvis and ureter.

Answer Key: a. Renal artery, b. Hilum, c. Renal vein, d. Renal pelvis, e. Ureter, f. Renal capsule, g. Major calyces, h. Renal sinus, i. Renal cortex, j. Renal pyramid (in renal medulla), k. Papilla, l. Renal column, m. Minor calyces, n. Segmental arteries, o. Interlobar artery, p. Interlobular artery, q. Arcuate arteries

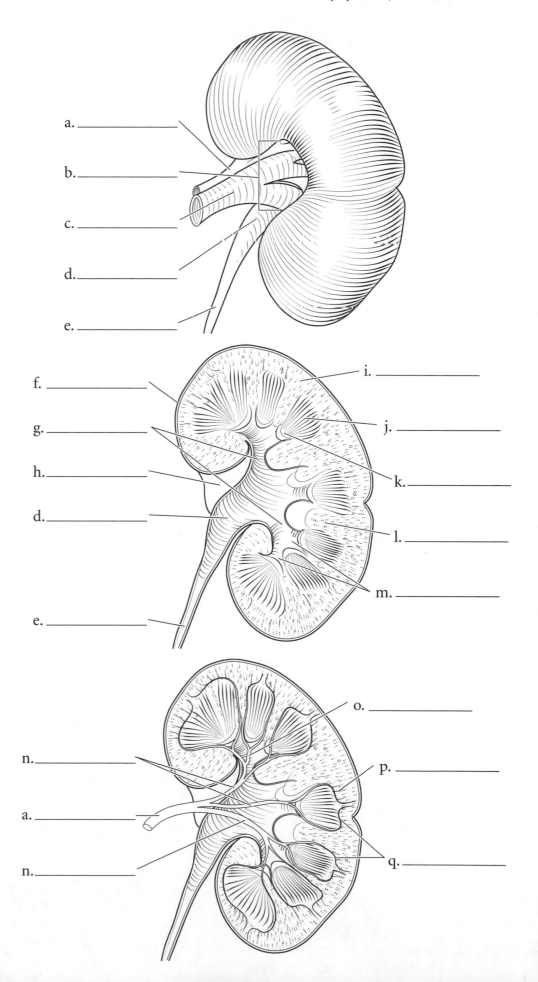

URINARY BLADDER

The **urinary bladder** is a storage organ for holding urine. The **ureters** enter the bladder at the **ureteral orifices** and the urethra exits the bladder inferiorly. These three openings make a triangular region known as the **trigone** at the posterior wall of the bladder. The **urethra** is the external tube that takes urine voided from the urinary bladder to outside the body. The urethra in the female is much shorter than in the male, which makes females more susceptible to bladder infections. The wall of the bladder consists of **smooth muscle** called the **detrusor muscle** and an inner lining of transitional epithelium. Label the features of the bladder, urethra, and associated structures and color them in.

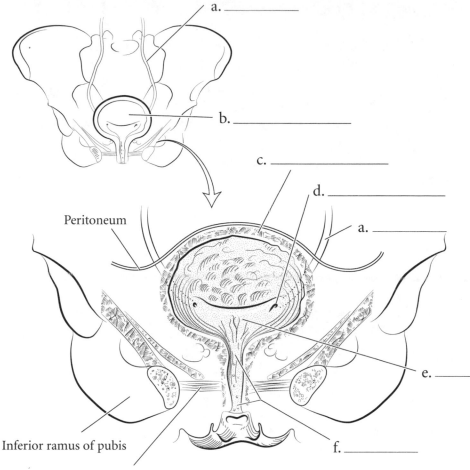

a. _____

b. _____

c. _____

d. _____

a. _____

Peritoneum

e. _____

Inferior ramus of pubis

f. _____

Urethral sphincter muscle

Female Urinary System

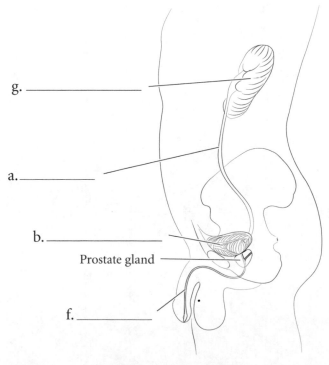

g. _____

a. _____

b. _____

Prostate gland

f. _____

Male Urinary System

Answer Key: a. Ureter, b. Urinary bladder, c. Detrusor muscle, d. Ureteral orifice, e. Trigone, f. Urethra, g. Right kidney

THE NEPHRON

The functional unit of the kidney is the **nephron**. It is here that material is filtered from the blood; some material is lost in the urine while other material is reabsorbed back into the cardiovascular system. The **renal corpuscle** of the nephron includes the **glomerulus** and the **glomerular (Bowman's) capsule**. The lining of the capsule wraps around the glomerulus and filtered material enters the nephron at this point. The glomerular capsule leads to the **proximal convoluted tubule**. This tubule has a brush border consisting of many microvilli and it provides for a great surface area for reabsorption of materials. Most of the reabsorption of material in the nephron occurs here. The peritubular capillaries wrap around the kidney tubules and reabsorb the filtered material. From the proximal convoluted tubule, the fluid flows into the **nephron loop (loop of Henle)**. The nephron loop takes fluid to the **distal convoluted tubule**. From here the filtrate flows into a **collecting duct**. Collecting ducts receive fluid from many nephrons. Label the parts of the nephron and associated structures and color them in. Each part of the nephron should be colored a different color.

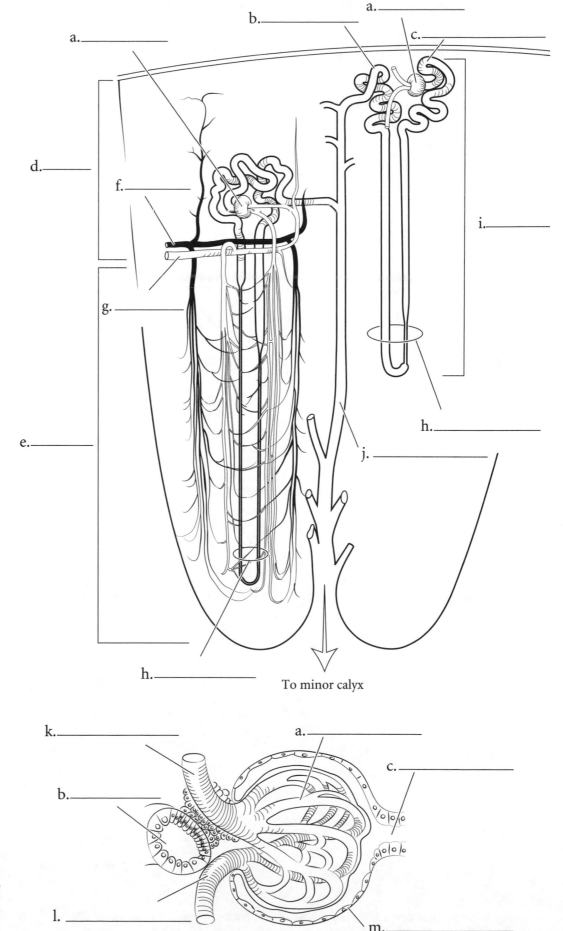

To minor calyx

Answer Key: a. Glomerulus, b. Distal convoluted tubule, c. Proximal convoluted tubule, d. Cortex, e. Medulla, f. Arcuate vein, g. Arcuate artery, h. Nephron loop (loop of Henle), i. Nephron, j. Collecting duct, k. Afferent arteriole, l. Efferent arteriole, m. Glomerular (Bowman's) capsule

OVERVIEW OF THE MALE REPRODUCTIVE SYSTEM

The male reproductive system consists of the two **testes**, the **epididymis**, the **ductus deferens** enclosed in the spermatic cord, the **seminal vesicles**, the **prostate** gland, the **bulbourethral glands**, and the **penis**. The testes are the glands that produce testosterone and sperm cells. Sperm cells travel from the testes to the epididymis where they are stored and mature. From the epididymis sperm cells move into the ductus deferens, which enters the body and travels to the posterior bladder.

From here the ductus deferens turns into the ejaculatory duct, which receives fluid from the semimal vesicles. The ejaculatory duct leads to the urethra where secretions from the prostate and bulbourethral glands are added. Finally the sperm cells and seminal fluid (together these make semen) are ejaculated from the penis.

Label the parts of the male reproductive system and color the various structures in the illustration.

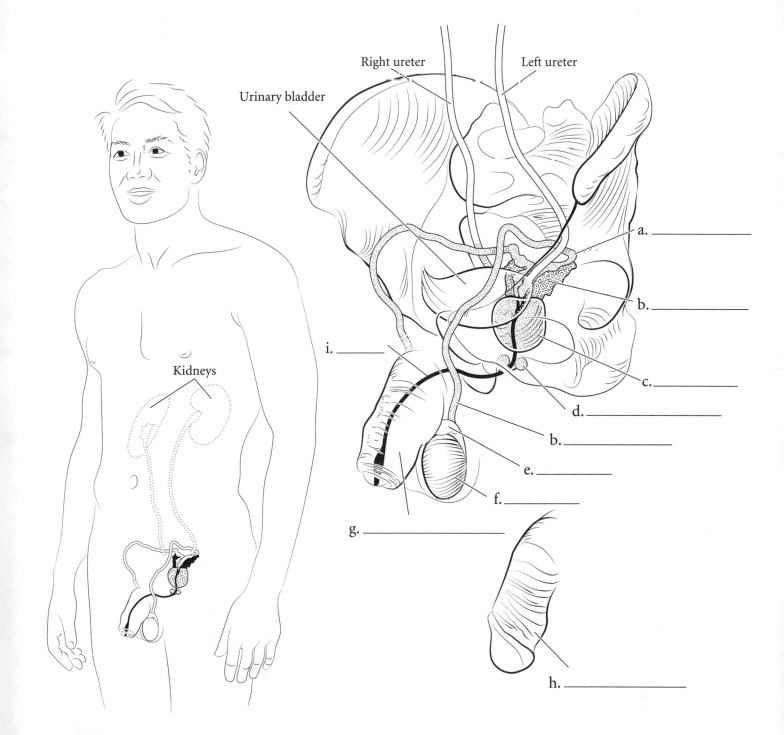

ORGANS OF THE MALE REPRODUCTIVE SYSTEM

The **testes** are enclosed in the **scrotal sac** which is lined with a smooth muscle layer called the **dartos muscle**. This muscle contracts when the temperatures drop near the testes, causing them to withdraw closer to the body where it is warmer. Another muscle of the region is the **cremaster muscle**. It also contracts when it is cold but it is made of skeletal muscle. The **epididymis** sits on top of the testis like a small cap and is a place where sperm cells mature. The **spermatic cord** consists of the cremaster muscle, the **ductus deferens**, the **testicular artery**, and a complex meshwork of veins called the **pampiniform plexus**. This plexus cools arterial blood flowing to the testes maintaining the testes at about 35 degrees C which is important for proper sperm maturation.

The sperm are produced in the seminiferous tubules of the testis. This occurs in **lobules of the testis** before they move to the epididymis. The epididymis has a series of long coiled tubules called the **ductus epididymis** and the sperm cells slowly pass through this ductwork. After the sperm cells mature in the epididymis they then travel to the **ductus deferens** which loops around the **ureters** before reaching the **seminal vesicles** located on the posterior surface of the **urinary bladder**. The seminal vesicles add a fluid that has buffers and that provides fructose to the sperm cells. From the seminal vesicles the fluid passes through the **ejaculatory duct** to the **prostate**. The prostate adds further fluid that is rich in buffers. This fluid passes into the urethra. The bulbourethral glands add a protein lubricant to the fluid. Label the organs and their features in the illustration and color them in different colors.

Answer Key: a. Ductus deferens, b. Pampiniform plexus, c. Testicular artery, d. Epididymis, e. Testis, f. Cremaster muscle and fascia, g. Scrotal skin and dartos muscle, h. Ureter, i. Urinary bladder, j. Seminal vesicle, k. Ejaculatory duct, l. Prostate, m. Bulbourethral gland, n. Urethra, o. Ductus epididymis, p. Lobules of testis

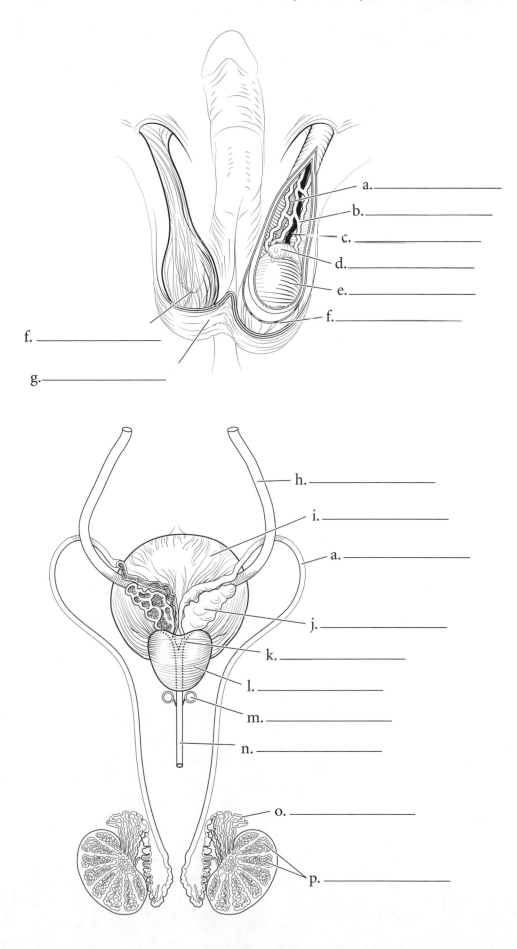

MIDSAGITTAL SECTION OF PELVIS/CROSS SECTION OF PENIS AND SEMINIFEROUS TUBULES

When seen in a midsagittal section, the relationship of the glands that produce seminal fluid can easily be seen. The **prostate** is approximately the size of a golf ball and is located inferior to the urinary bladder. The prostatic urethra is the portion of the urethra that is enclosed in the prostate. The **bulbourethral glands** are located in the wall of the pelvic floor and the **seminal vesicles** are posterior to the urinary bladder. Exterior to the body wall are the testes and these are enclosed in the **scrotal sac**. The **epididymis** receives sperm from the testis and has three parts, a **head**, a **body**, and a **tail**. The **symphysis pubis** is an important reference point in the midsagittal section. In males there is a flap of tissue encircling the **glans penis**. This is the **prepuce** (foreskin) and it is sometimes removed at birth in a procedure called a circumcision. The **corpus cavernosum** can be seen in this section along with the **corpus spongiosum** and the **spongy urethra**.

The cross section of the penis illustrates the relative position of the erectile tissue in the male. On the dorsal aspect of the penis are the paired **corpora cavernosa** (*corpus cavernosum* singular). These cylinders fill with blood and produce an increase in length and diameter of the penis. These, along with the **corpus spongiosum**, are involved in making the penis erect. The corpus spongiosum contains the **spongy urethra**. The **deep dorsal vein** of the penis is also seen in cross section. Label the structures seen in a cross section of the penis and color in the erectile tissue and the spongy urethra.

The formation of sperm is known as spermatogenesis and occurs from **spermatogonia** on the superficial wall of the seminiferous tubules. These produce cells called **primary spermatocytes** which in turn mature into **secondary spermatocytes**. **Spermatids** derive from secondary spermatocytes and they, in turn, become **spermatozoa** (sperm cells). **Sertoli cells** assist in the process. Label the cells and color each one in a separate color.

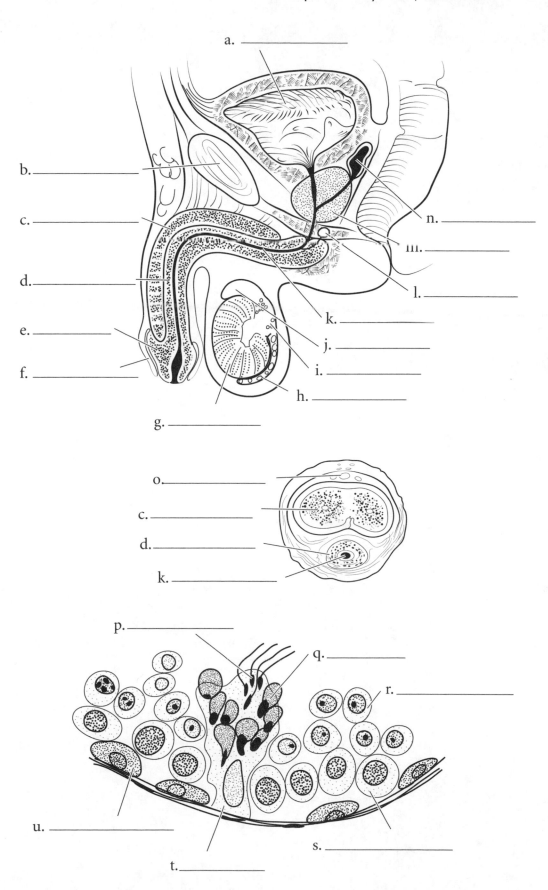

Answer Key: a. Urinary bladder, b. Symphysis pubis, c. Corpus cavernosum, d. Corpus spongiosum, e. Glans penis, f. Prepuce, g. Testis, h. Tail of epididymis, i. Body of epididymis, j. Head of epididymis, k. Spongy urethra, l. Bulbourethral gland, m. Prostate, n. Seminal vesicle, o. Deep dorsal vein, p. Spermatozoa, q. Spermatids, r. Secondary spermatocytes, s. Primary spermatocytes, t. Sertoli cell, u. Spermatogonia

OVERVIEW OF THE FEMALE REPRODUCTIVE SYSTEM

The female reproductive system consists of the two **ovaries**, the **uterine tubes**, a single **uterus**, **vagina**, and the **vaginal orifice**. The uterus is held to the anterior body by the round ligaments and held to the pelvic wall by the suspensory ligaments. Blood flows to the ovaries by the **gonadal arteries**.

The breasts are integumentary structures and each one has **mammary glands**, the **areola**, and the **nipple**. Label the structures of the female reproductive system and color each of them in a different color.

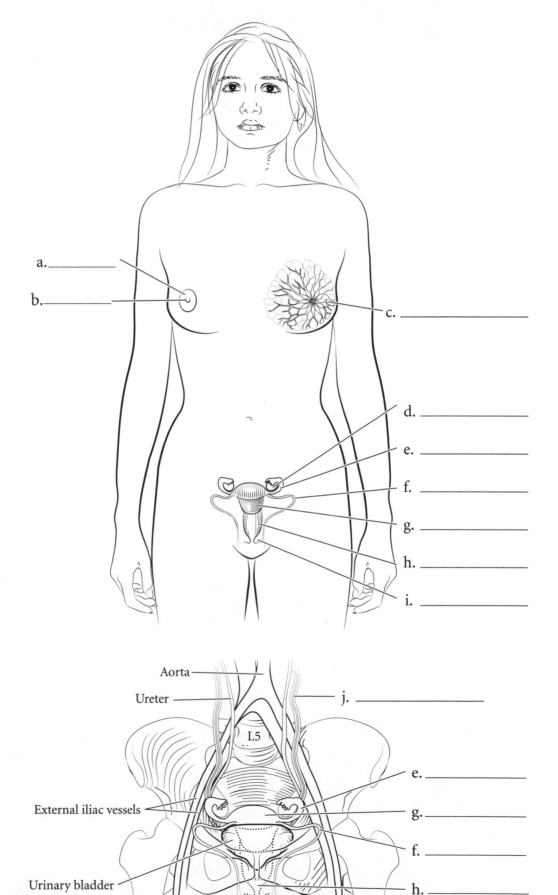

a. _____

b. _____

c. _____

d. _____

e. _____

f. _____

g. _____

h. _____

i. _____

Aorta

Ureter

j. _____

L5

External iliac vessels

e. _____

g. _____

f. _____

Urinary bladder

h. _____

Answer Key: a. Areola, b. Nipple, c. Mammary glands, d. Ovary, e. Uterine tube, f. Round ligament, g. Uterus, h. Vagina, i. Labium minus, j. Ovarian vessels

MIDSAGITTAL

The **ovaries** produce the oocytes that are released into the pelvic cavity. Locate the **suspensory ligaments** that attach the ovaries to the pelvic wall. The **round ligament** attaches the uterus anteriorly. The oocytes travel into the **uterine tubes** and then pass into the **uterus**. The uterus has a domed **fundus** near the entrance of the uterine tubes and a **cervix** that inserts into the vagina. The depression between the uterus and the rectum is the **rectouterine pouch**. The **vagina** is inferior to the uterus and terminates with the vaginal orifice. Anterior to the vaginal orifice is the urethral orifice, the external opening of the urethra. In this section

you can see the fornix of the vagina, a pocket that surrounds the cervix of the uterus. You can also see the relationship of the **labium minus** and the **labium majus** in this section. The labia minora are the inner vaginal lips and the labia majora are the outer vaginal lips. These are part of the vulva or external genitalia. Another part of the vulva is the **clitoris** which consists of the external glans and the body of the clitoris. The body of the clitoris is imbedded in the body tissue. The glans is covered with a prepuce. Anterior to the clitoris is the mons pubis, a fatty pad of tissue overlying the symphysis pubis. Label the organs and other structures in the midsagittal section of the female pelvis and color the structures in using different colors for each structure or space.

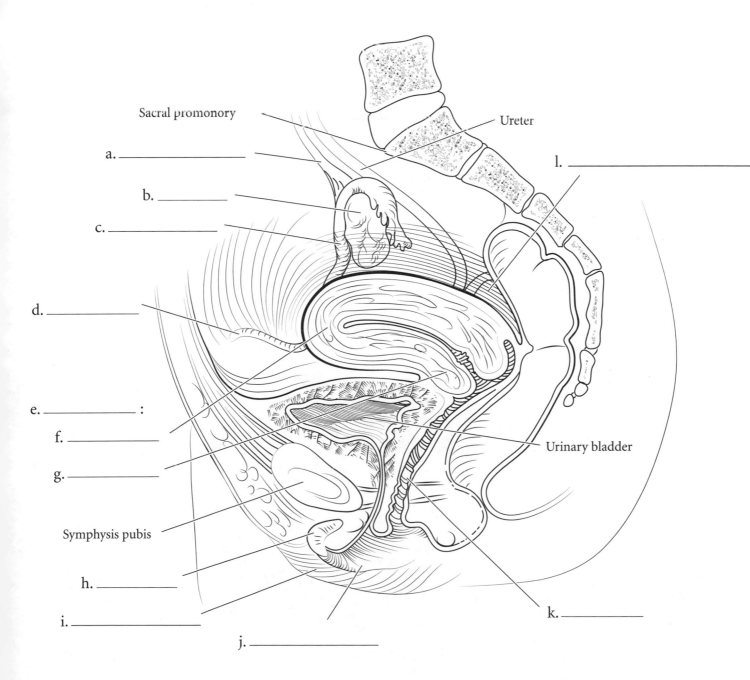

Sacral promonory

Ureter

a. _____

b. _____

c. _____

l. _____

d. _____

e. _____ :

f. _____

g. _____

Urinary bladder

Symphysis pubis

h. _____

i. _____

j. _____

k. _____

Answer Key: a. Suspensory ligaments, b. Ovary, c. Uterine tube, d. Round ligament, e. Uterus, f. Fundus, g. Cervix, h. Clitoris, i. Labium majus, j. Labium minus, k. Vagina, l. Rectouterine pouch

OVARY

The **ovary** is the gonad of the female reproductive system. The background tissue of the ovary is called the stroma. It produces **oocytes** in a process known as oogenesis and when they are mature they are released from the ovary by ovulation. The ovary has **primordial follicles** that contain **primary oocytes**. When the primary oocytes get a little larger they are located in **primary follicles**. As the ovulatory cycle progresses some of these primary oocytes develop into **secondary oocytes**. These are enclosed in **secondary follicles**. Usually only one of these oocytes enlarges and is ovulated.

There are two cycles that occur in the female reproductive system and they are interrelated. The **ovarian cycle** involves the maturation of the oocytes, ovulation, and the development of the **corpus luteum**. This cycle can be divided into the **preovulatory phase**, **ovulation**, and the **postovulatory phase**. The **menstrual cycle** involves the changes in the endometrium. The endometrium has a **basal layer** that stays the same thickness during the menstrual cycle and a **functional layer** that grows larger in the early part of the menstrual cycle, becomes rich in glycogen during the middle of a woman's cycle, and then is shed during menstruation.

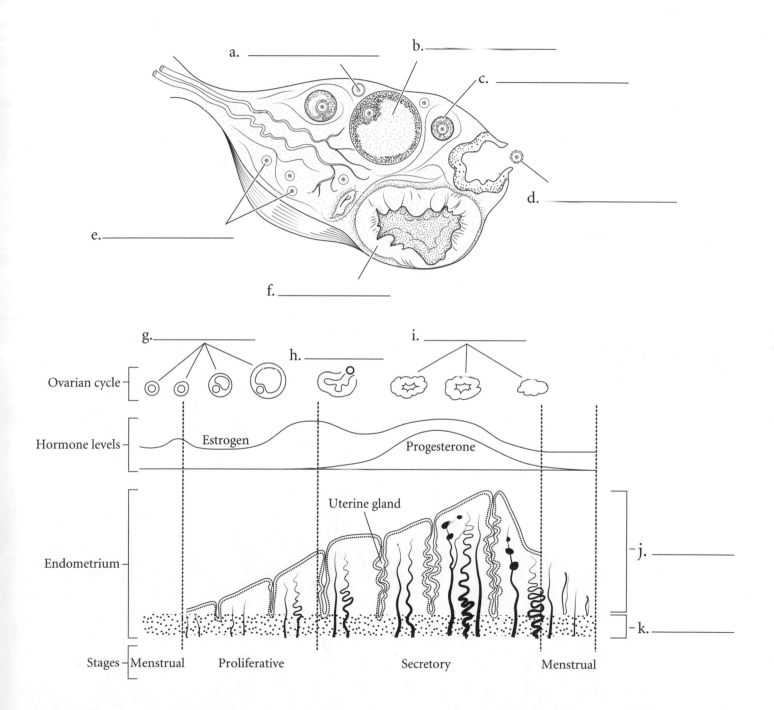

Answer Key: a. Primary oocytes, b. Secondary follicles, c. Primary follicle, d. Secondary oocytes, e. Primordial follicles, f. Corpus luteum, g. Preovulatory phase, h. Ovulation, i. Postovulatory phase, j. Functional layer, k. Basal layer

SECTION OF UTERUS AND VAGINA

The **oocyte** is ovulated from the **ovary** and moves into the **uterine tube**. The uterine tube is fringed by small cylindrical structures called **fimbriae**. The **uterus** is a small, flask-shaped organ. The uterus has a domed **fundus**, a main **body,** a narrowed **isthmus**, and an inferior **cervix**. The **uterosacral ligament** attaches the uterus to the sacrum. Most of the uterine wall is made of the myometrium which is a thick layer of smooth muscle. The **vagina** is approximately ten centimeters in length and is lined with stratified squamous epithelium and smooth muscle. A small ring of mucous membrane called the **hymen** is present in the vagina and is frequently torn during first intercourse. The hymen can rupture prior to intercourse and is not a good indicator of virginity. The vagina has **rugae** which are folds in the vaginal wall. These stimulate the penis and also allow for expansion of the vagina during delivery. Label the **suspensory ligament** and **ovarian ligament** as well as the structures of the uterus, ovary, and vagina. Color the regions of the uterus, ovary, vagina, and associated structures.

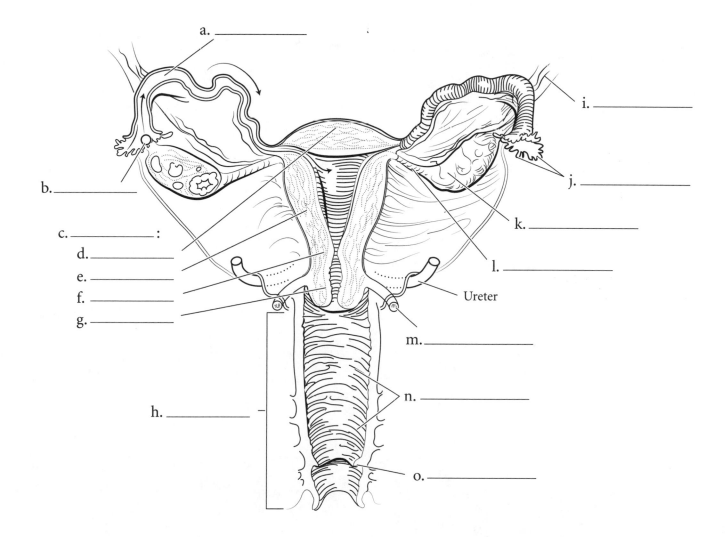

a. _____

i. _____

b. _____

j. _____

c. _____ :

k. _____

d. _____

e. _____

l. _____

f. _____

Ureter

g. _____

m. _____

n. _____

h. _____

o. _____

Answer Key: a. Uterine tube, b. Oocyte, c. Uterus, d. Fundus, e. Body, f. Isthmus, g. Cervix, h. Vagina, i. Suspensory ligament, j. Fimbriae, k. Ovary, l. Ovarian ligament, m. Uterosacral ligament. n. Rugae, o. Hymen

FEMALE BREAST AND EXTERNAL GENITALIA

The **mammary glands** are located in the breast. They produce milk when a woman is lactating and lead to **lactiferous ducts**. These ducts take milk to the **lactiferous sinuses** which drain into the nipple. Because breast cancer is a significant cause of mortality in women, the lymph drainage of the breast is important. Primary tumors may originate in the breast tissue and then migrate by **lymphatic vessels** to the **axillary lymph nodes**. This is one of the main ways that breast cancer spreads. There is a small series of **parasternal lymph nodes** that takes a small portion of the lymph back to the cardiovascular system.

The floor of the pelvis is known as the perineum and can be divided into a **urogenital triangle** and an **anal triangle**. The anal triangle contains the **anus** and the urogenital triangle houses the **vaginal orifice**, the **urethral orifice**, and the **clitoris**. The **mons pubis** is the most anterior part of the external genitalia and posterior to that is the **prepuce**. This structure envelops the **clitoris**. The **labia majora** and the **labia minora** encircle the **vaginal orifice**. The vagina is lubricated internally by some glands during arousal and intercourse as well as from the greater vestibular glands located laterally and posteriorly to the vaginal orifice. Label the structures of the female breast and the external genitalia and color them in.

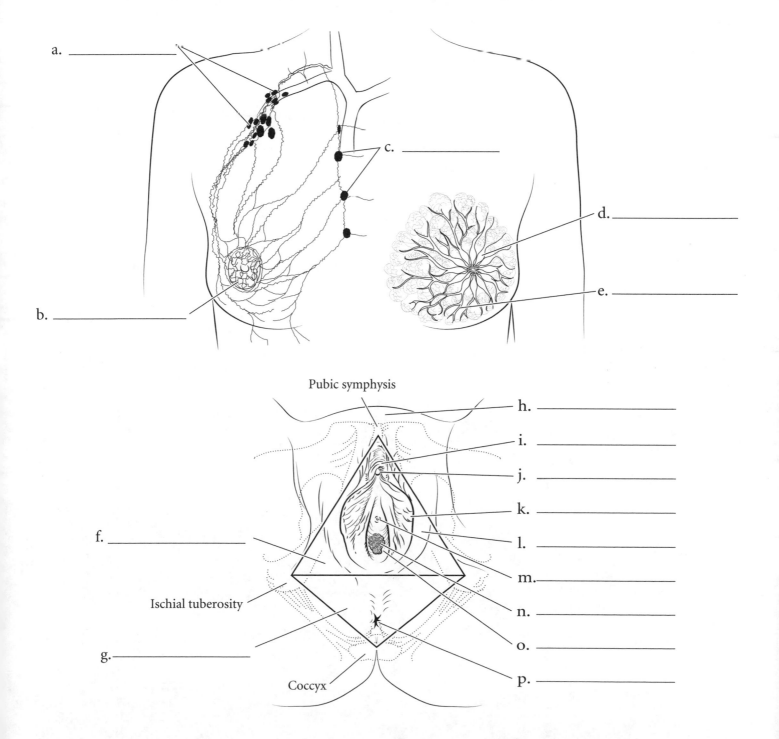

a. _____
b. _____
c. _____
d. _____
e. _____

Pubic symphysis

Ischial tuberosity

Coccyx

f. _____
g. _____
h. _____
i. _____
j. _____
k. _____
l. _____
m. _____
n. _____
o. _____
p. _____

Answer Key: a. Axillary lymph nodes, b. Lymphatic vessels, c. Parasternal lymph nodes, d. Lactiferous sinuses, e. Lactiferous ducts, f. Urogenital triangle, g. Anal triangle, h. Mons pubis, i. Prepuce, j. Clitoris, k. Labia minora, l. Labia majora, m. Urethral orifice, n. Vaginal orifice, o. Greater vestibular gland, p. Anus

PREEMBRYONIC STAGE

The process of development begins with the union of the sperm and oocyte. After **ovulation**, the secondary oocyte moves down the uterine tube and, if **fertilization** occurs by sperm, it usually happens in the uterine tube. Once fertilization occurs, the oocyte and the sperm unite to become a **zygote**. The zygote divides during this **preembryonic stage** and forms a **two-celled stage**. These cells go through numerous divisions and are called **blastomeres**. The two blastomeres divide and become four cells and this process continues until a cluster of cells

(16 to 32 of them) is formed called a **morula**. As division continues this cluster becomes a hollow ball of cells called a **blastocyst**. The hollow cavity of the blastocyst is called the **blastocele** and most of the wall of the blastocyst consists of a layer of simple squamous epithelia called the **trophoblast**. One part of the wall consists of an inner cell mass known as the **embryoblast**. Some of these cells will develop into the embryo. Label the structures in the preembryonic stage of development. Color in the various stages in different colors and use one color for the trophoblast and another for the embryoblast.

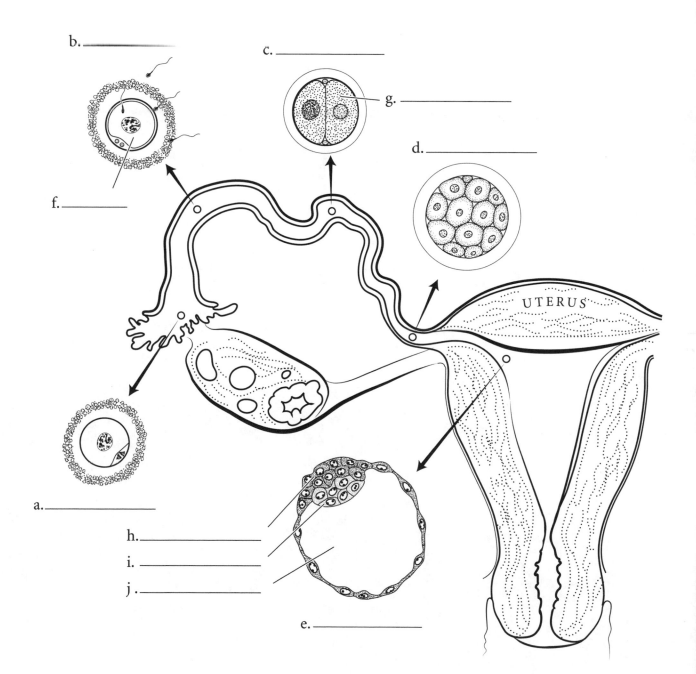

b. _____
c. _____
g. _____
d. _____
f. _____
a. _____
h. _____
i. _____
j. _____
e. _____

UTERUS

Answer Key: a. Ovulation, b. Fertilization, c. Two-cell stage, d. Morula, e. Blastocyst, f. Zygote, g. Blastomere, h. Trophoblast, i. Embryoblast, j. Blastocele

EMBRYONIC STAGE

The blastocyst is the stage of development in which implantation in the uterus occurs. Implantation is the imbedding of the blastocyst in the endometrium of the mother. Once this occurs, a hollow space develops in the embryoblast and this is called the **amniotic cavity**. At this time, the embryoblast is divided into a **bilaminar germ disk** with two primitive tissues called the **epiblast** and the **hypoblast**. The **primitive streak** forms along the anterior/posterior axis of the embryo and it becomes a region of growth in the early stage of development.

From the epiblast the embryoblast begins to form three primary germ layers. These are the **endoderm**, **ectoderm**, and **mesoderm**. The structure is now referred to as a **trilaminar germ disk** (meaning a developmental structure with three layers). The development of the **notochord** begins and this structure will make up the center part (nucleosus pulposus) of the intervertebral disks in the adult. The **yolk sac** also forms during this period. Once the germ layers are formed, the preembryonic stage ends and the developing tissue is known as an embryo. The embryonic stage begins about day 16 after fertilization and lasts until about the eighth week of pregnancy. During the embryonic stage, the major organs of the body are initiated in a process called organogenesis.

During the first part of the embryonic phase, the ectoderm begins to fold in on itself and becomes a **neural groove**. This will develop into the nervous system of the body. Other derivatives of the ectoderm are the epidermis and some of the facial bones and muscles. The mesoderm gives rise to most of the bones and muscles of the body, the dermis, and the circulatory system. The endodermis gives rise to the linings of the gastrointestinal tract and respiratory system, and some glands. As development continues, the neural groove folds in on itself and becomes a **neural tube** and the formation of the **gut** takes place. Label the structures in the embryonic phase and use blue colors for the ectoderm and derivatives of the ectoderm such as the neural tissue. Use red for the mesoderm and color the endoderm in yellow.

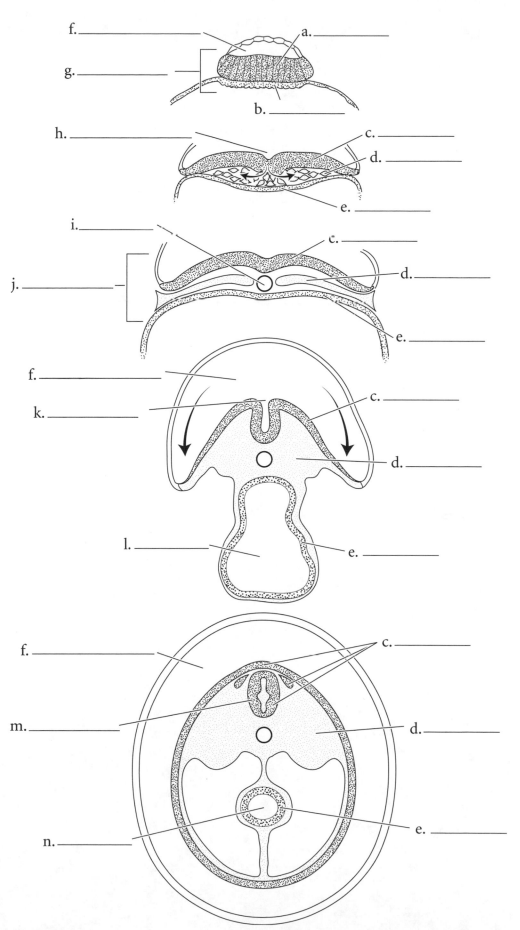

Answer Key: a. Epiblast, b. Hypoblast, c. Ectoderm, d. Mesoderm, e. Endoderm, f. Amniotic cavity, g. Bilaminar germ disk, h. Primitive streak, i. Notochord, j. Trilaminar germ disk, k. Neural groove, l. Yolk sac, m. Neural tube, n. Gut

FETAL STAGE

At the eighth week after fertilization the organs are formed and the embryo has now become a **fetus**. Prior to the fetal stage the outer wall of the **embryo** develops into a membrane called the **chorion** and some of this membrane is joined with the maternal vasculature and forming the **placenta**. Between the chorion and the embryo is the **chorionic cavity**. This cavity disappears by the eighth week. A membrane called the **amnion** folds around the embryo forming the **amniotic cavity** and this cavity is filled with amnitoic fluid.

The stages of development can be divided into the pre-embryo (from fertilization to two weeks), the embryo (up to eight weeks after fertilization) and the final stage, the fetus (after eight weeks). The conceptus is the term used for the developing cells and tissues from the pre-embryo through the fetus.

Before delivery of the fetus, the amniotic sac ruptures releasing amniotic fluid, the uterus contracts expelling the fetus from the uterus, and the final stage occurs when the placenta is released.

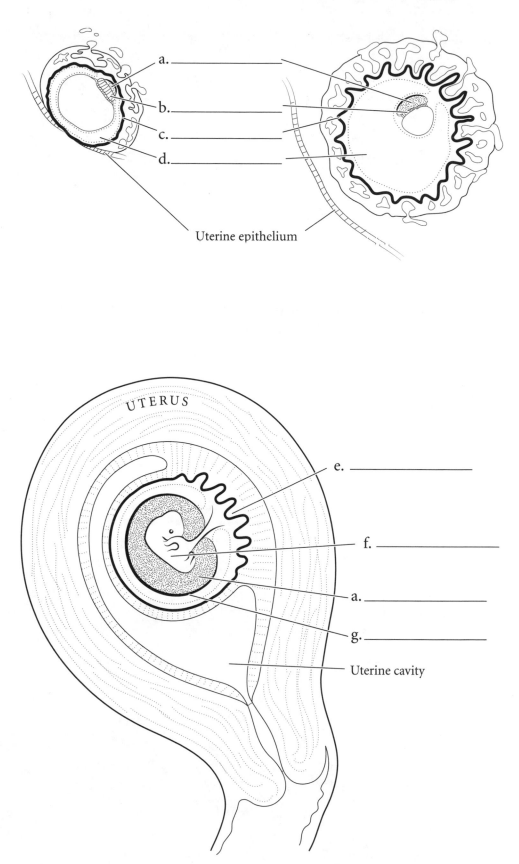

a. _____
b. _____
c. _____
d. _____

Uterine epithelium

UTERUS

e. _____
f. _____
a. _____
g. _____

Uterine cavity

Answer Key: a. Amniotic cavity, b. Embryo, c. Chorion, d. Chorionic cavity, e. Placenta, f. Fetus, g. Amnion

articular cartilages, 89

articular disc, 95

articular facet, 55, 57

articular process, 57, 59

articulate artery, 215

articulations, 85–101

arytenoid cartilages, 259

astrocytes, 107

atlas, 55

atom, 5

atrioventricular bundle, 203

atrioventricular node, 203

atrium, 193, 201

auditory association area, 125

auditory canal, 167

auditory cortex, 125

auditory tube (Eustachian tube), 167, 169

auricle (pinna), 167

auricular surface, 59

auricular vein, 225

autonomic nervous system, 103, 149, 151

axillary artery, 207, 213

axillary lymph nodes, 309

axillary nerve, 141

axillary vein, 223, 227

axis, 55

axon hillcock, 105

axons, 37, 105, 107

azygos veins, 231

B

B cells, 195, 247

ball and socket joints, 91

basal layer, 305

basal nuclei, 121

basement membrane, 23, 255

basilar artery, 211

basilar membrane, 173

basilic vein, 223, 227

basophilic cells, 177

basophils, 195

bicuspid valve, 201, 203

bicuspids (premolars), 273

bifid spinous process, 57

bilaminar germ disk, 313

bile canaliculi, 283

bile duct, 283, 285

bipolar layer, 165

bipolar neurons, 109

bladder, 13

  gall, 267, 279, 285

  urinary, 287, 291, 297

blastocele, 311

blastocyst, 311

blastomeres, 311

blood, 35, 195

blood vessels, 13, 165, 205, 273

body cavities, 19

body regions, 15, 17

bolus, 275

bone(s), 35

  forearm, 71

  frontal, 43, 45, 47

  hand, 73

  hyoid, 259

  lacrimal, 45

  nasal, 43, 45, 253, 255

  occipital, 45, 47

  palatine, 47, 49

  parietal, 45, 47

  pisiform, 73

  sphenoid, 43, 45, 47, 51, 177

  tarsal, 83

  temporal, 43, 45, 51

  zygomatic, 43

bony labryinth, 171

border, medial, 65

bound ribosomes, 21

Bowman's capsule, 293

brachial artery, 191, 207, 213

brachial plexus, 137, 141

brachial region, 15, 17

brachial veins, 223, 227

brachiocephalic artery, 209

brachiocephalic trunk, 207

brachiocephalic veins, 223, 225

brain, 9, 103, 113, 115, 117, 119, 121

brain arteries, 211

breast, female, 309

Broca's area, 125

bronchi, 251, 265

bronchial tree, 261, 265

bronchioles, 265

bronchus, 261

bulbourethral glands, 295, 299

bundle branches, 203

bursa, 89

C

calcaneal region, 17

calcaneus, 83

calyces, 289

capillaries, 193, 205, 235, 245, 265

capitate, 73

capitulum, 69

carbohydrate chains, 21

cardia, 277

cardiac muscle, 37

cardiac notch, 263

cardiac vein, 197, 199

cardiovascular system, 13, 191–234

carina, 261

carnucle, 159

carotid artery, 191, 207, 209, 211

INTRODUCTION

Muscles can be grouped into anatomical regions such as muscles of the head, arm or torso. Muscles can also be functionally related, for example, muscles that act on the thigh or muscles that flex the hand.

Origin, Insertion, Action

The **origin** of the muscle is the stable part of the muscle. The majority of muscles have origins that are superior, proximal, or medial to the insertion. There are only a few exceptions to this rule. The **insertion** of the muscle is the part of the muscle that has the greatest motion when the muscle contracts. In some cases a muscle can move either the origin or the insertion and you should learn the origins and insertions as presented. The **action** of a muscle is what the muscle does. Some muscles are flexors and decrease joint angles. Some are extensors, adductors, abductors, rotators, etc. The action of the muscle is every movement the muscle does.

When you study muscles, it helps to take two or three at a time and learn just the origins of the muscles. When you know those, then study the insertions, and finally, the actions. After you know the muscles well, then take another group of muscles and add them to the list. If you try to learn twenty muscles at a time, the task will be frustrating, so it is best to take them in small groups.

Muscle Names

The muscles are named by different criteria and understanding how they are named can help you to remember the muscle. Muscles can be named for their shape. The *trapezius* is a trapezoid-like muscle. The *rhomboideus* muscles are shaped like a rhombus. Muscles can be named by the number of heads they have. The *triceps* brachii has three heads. Muscles can be named by location. The *rectus abdominis* literally means "the straight muscle of the abdomen." The *tibialis anterior* is the front muscle on the tibia. Muscles can be named according to size. The teres *major* is the large muscle and the teres *minor* is the small muscle. *Teres* means "round." Some muscles are superficial while others are deep. The flexor digitorum *superficialis* is superficial to the flexor digitorum *profundus*. Muscles can also be named for their action. There are the *adductors*, the *flexors* and *extensor* muscles, etc.

Muscles that cross joints of the body move those joints. The main muscle that causes the joint to move is called the **prime mover** or **agonist**. A muscle that helps the prime mover is called a **synergist**. A muscle that opposes the prime mover is called an **antagonist**. If both the prime mover and the antagonist contract, then the joint is **fixed**.

Muscle Groups

There are groups of muscles that act together. The **rotator cuff** (**musculotendinous cuff**) muscles stabilize the shoulder joint. These are the supraspinatus, the infraspinatus the teres minor and the subscapularis. The **abdominal muscles** are the rectus abdominis, the external oblique, the internal oblique, and the transversus abdominis. The **quadriceps femoris** group are the muscles of the anterior thigh. These are the rectus femoris, the vastus lateralis, the vastus medialis, and the vastus intermedius. The **hamstrings** are muscles on the posterior thigh and they consist of the biceps femoris, the semitendinosus, and the semimembranosus. There are many more functional groups of muscles but these are a few of the major ones.

The muscles of the body are numerous and flash cards are a great tool to learn muscles. Cut out the cards along the lines. As we said before, it is best to take a few cards at a time and learn them well. You should color each muscle on the front side of the card and put a small 'O' where the origin of the muscle is and a small 'I" where the insertion of the muscle is. Each muscle is illustrated isolated from other muscles so that the origin and the insertion are plainly visible. The name of the muscle is on the back of the illustration. The origin (O), insertion (I), and action (A) are listed for each muscle on the back of the card.

MUSCLES, ANTERIOR VIEW

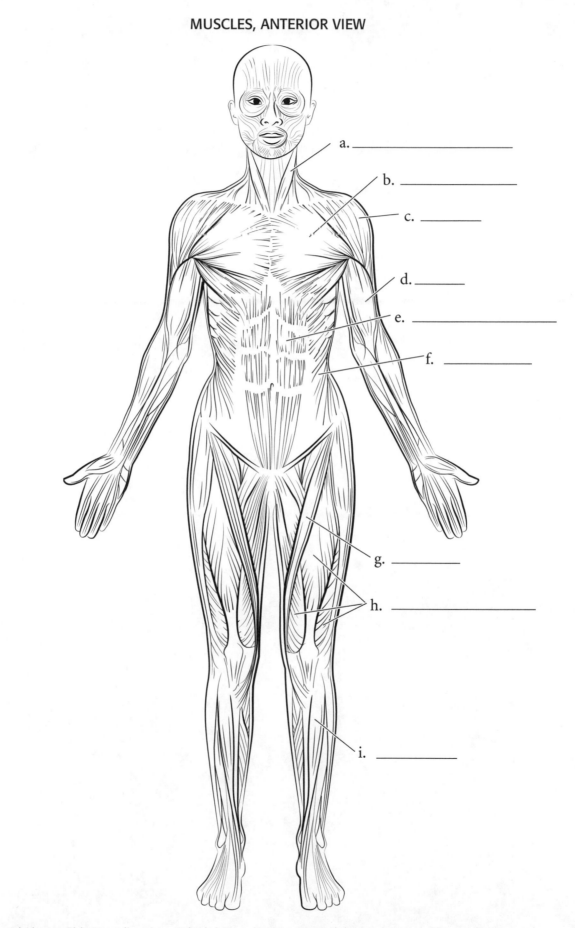

a. _____

b. _____

c. _____

d. _____

e. _____

f. _____

g. _____

h. _____

i. _____

Answer Key: a. Sternocleidomastoid, b. Pectoralis major, c. Deltoid, d. Biceps brachii, e. Rectus abdominis, f. External oblique, g. Sartorius, h. Quadriceps femoris, i. Tibialis anterior

MUSCLES, POSTERIOR VIEW

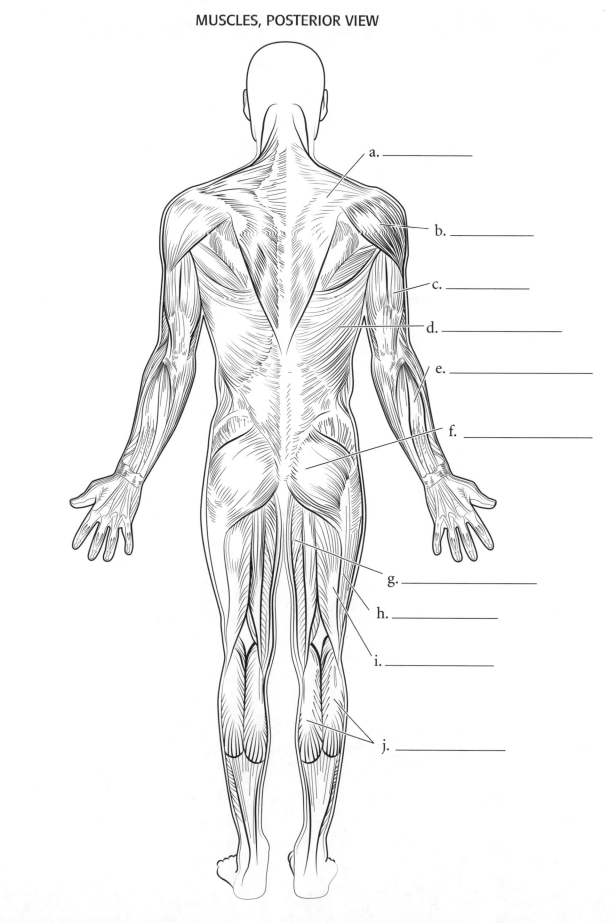

a. _____

b. _____

c. _____

d. _____

e. _____

f. _____

g. _____

h. _____

i. _____

j. _____

Answer Key: a. Trapezius, b. Deltoid, c.Triceps brachii, d. Latissimus dorsi, e. Extensor digitorum, f. Gluteus maximus, g. Adductor magnus, h. Iliotibial tract, i. Biceps femoris, j. Gastrocnemius

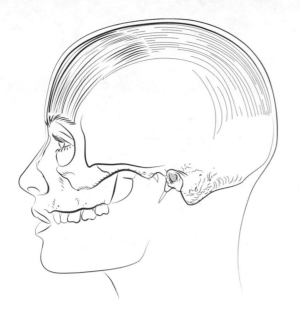
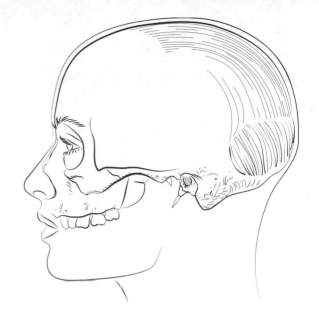
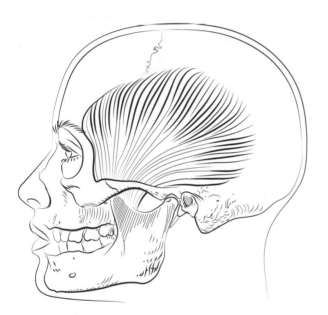
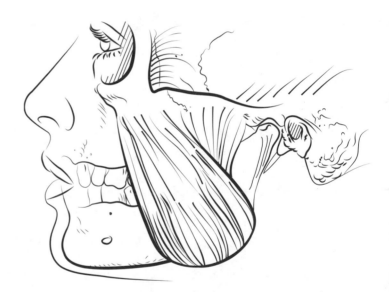
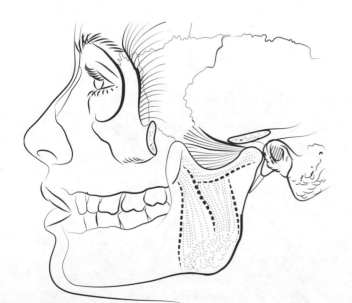
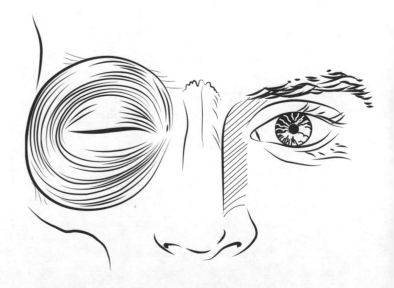

OCCIPITALIS

O: Occipital bone and temporal bone

I: Galea aponeurotica

A: Pulls scalp posteriorly

FRONTALIS

O: Galea aponeurotica

I: Skin near eyebrows

A: Raises eyebrows, pulls scalp anteriorly

MASSETER

O: Zygomatic arch

I: Ramus of mandible

A: Closes mandible

TEMPORALIS

O: Temporal fossa

I: Coronoid process and ramus of the mandible

A: Closes mandible

ORBICULARIS OCULI

O: Frontal bone and maxilla on medial orbit

I: Eyelid

A: Closes eye

MEDIAL AND LATERAL PTERYGOIDS

O: Pterygoid processes of sphenoid bone

I: Ramus and condylar process of mandible on medial side

A: Lateral movement of mandible

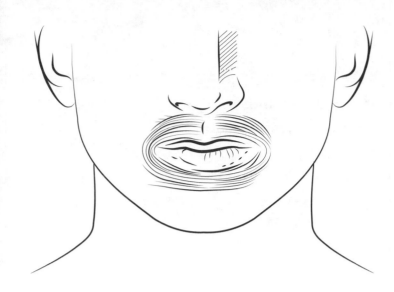
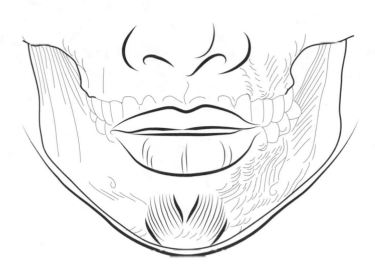
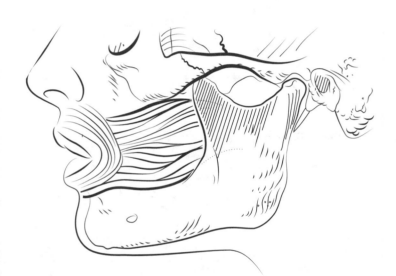
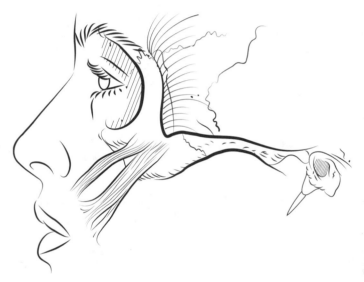
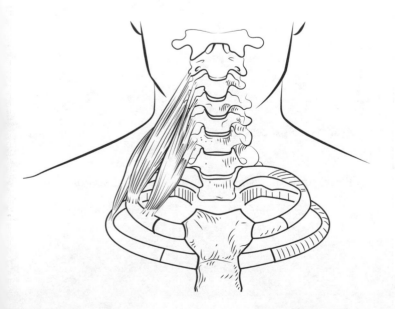
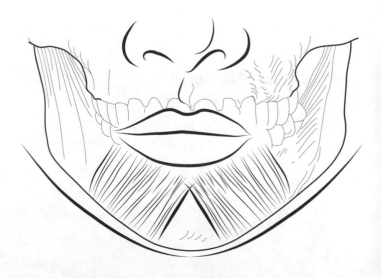

MENTALIS

O: Anterior, medial mandible

I: Skin of chin

A: Elevates lower lip

ORBICULARIS ORIS

O: Muscles encircling mouth

I: Skin of lips

A: Closes mouth

ZYGOMATICUS

O: Zygomatic bone

I: Angle of mouth

A: Elevates corners of mouth (in a smile or laugh)

BUCCINATOR

O: Mandible and maxilla

I: Orbicularis oris

A: Tightens cheek

DEPRESSOR LABII INFERIORIS

O: Inferior border of mandible

I: Skin of inferior lip, and orbicularis oris muscle

A: Depresses lower lip

SCALENUS

O: Transverse process of C 2–6

I: Ribs 1 and 2

A: Flexes and rotates neck, elevates first and second ribs

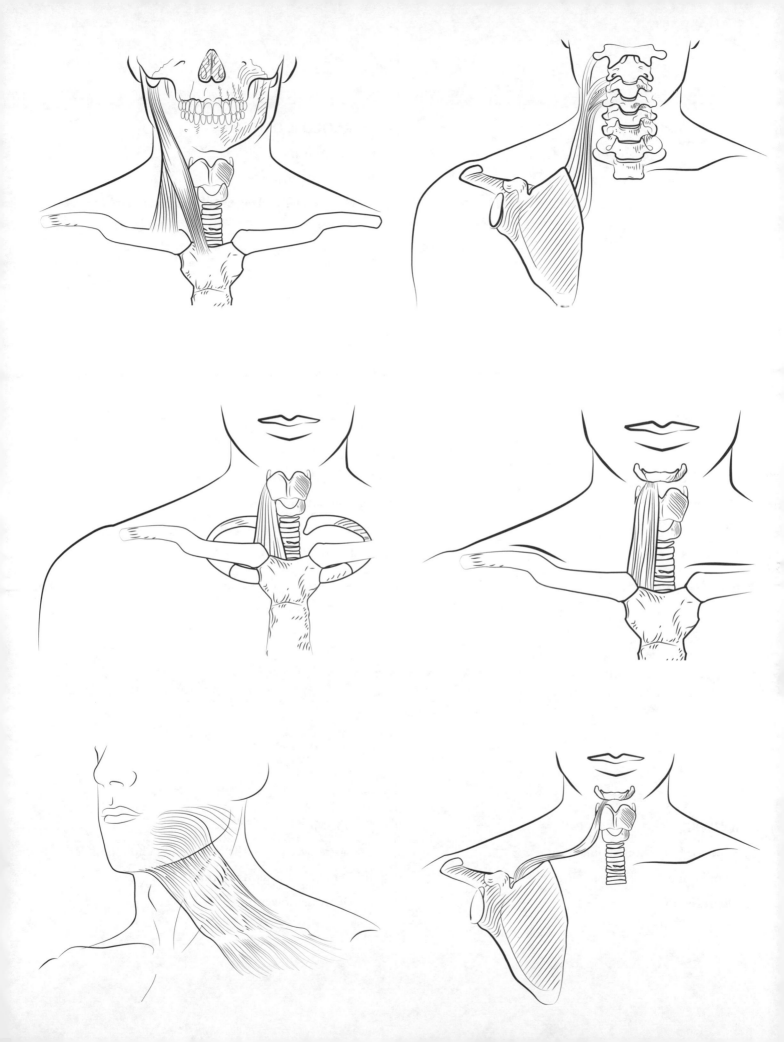

LEVATOR SCAPULAE

O: Transverse processes of C1–4

I: Superior angle of scapula

A: Elevates scapula, rotates and abducts neck

STERNOCLEIDOMASTOID

O: Sternum and clavicle

I: Mastoid process

A: One: rotates and extends head, both: flexes neck

STERNOHYOID

O: Manubrium of sternum

I: Hyoid bone

A: Depresses hyoid bone

STERNOTHYROID

O: Manubrium of sternum

I: Thyroid cartilage of larynx

A: Depresses thyroid cartilage

OMOHYOID

O: Superior border of scapula

I: Hyoid bone

A: Depresses hyoid

PLATYSMA

O: Fascia over pectoralis major and deltoid muscles

I: Mandible and skin inferior to lower lip

A: Depresses lower lip

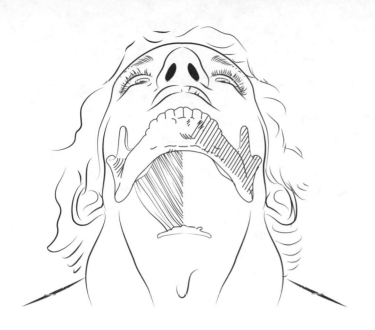
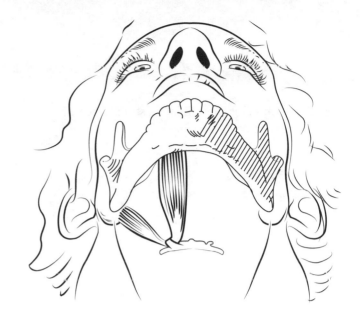
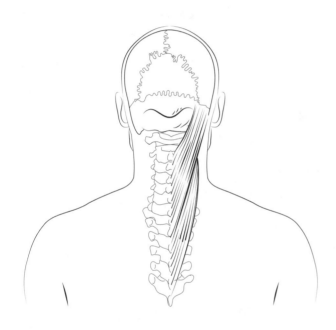
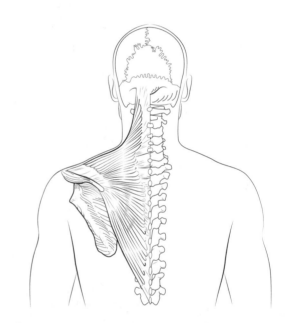
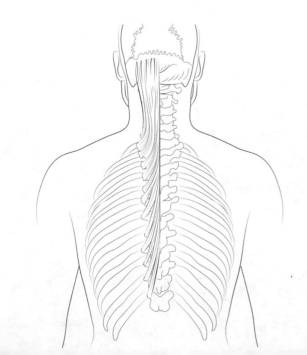
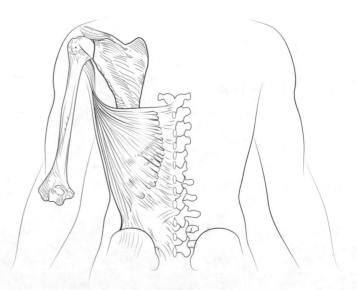

DIGASTRIC

O: Anterior, inferior mandible, mastoid notch of temporal bone

I: Hyoid bone

A: Protracts, retracts, and elevates hyoid, opens mandible

MYLOHYOID

O: Inner margin of mandible

I: Hyoid bone

A: Elevates floor of oral cavity

TRAPEZIUS

O: Occipital protuberance, ligamentum nuchae, C7–T12

I: Clavicle, acromion, and spine of scapula

A: Abducts and extends head, rotates and adducts scapula

SPLENIUS

O: Ligamentum nuchae, C7–T6

I: C2–4, occipital bone, temporal bone

A: Extends and rotates head

LATISSIMUS DORSI

O: T7–T12, L1–L5, sacrum, iliac crest, ribs 10–12

I: Intertubercular groove of humerus

A: Adducts, extends, and medially rotates arm, pulls shoulder inferiorly

SEMISPINALIS

O: C4–T12

I: Occipital bone, T1–4

A: Extends head, rotates vertebral column

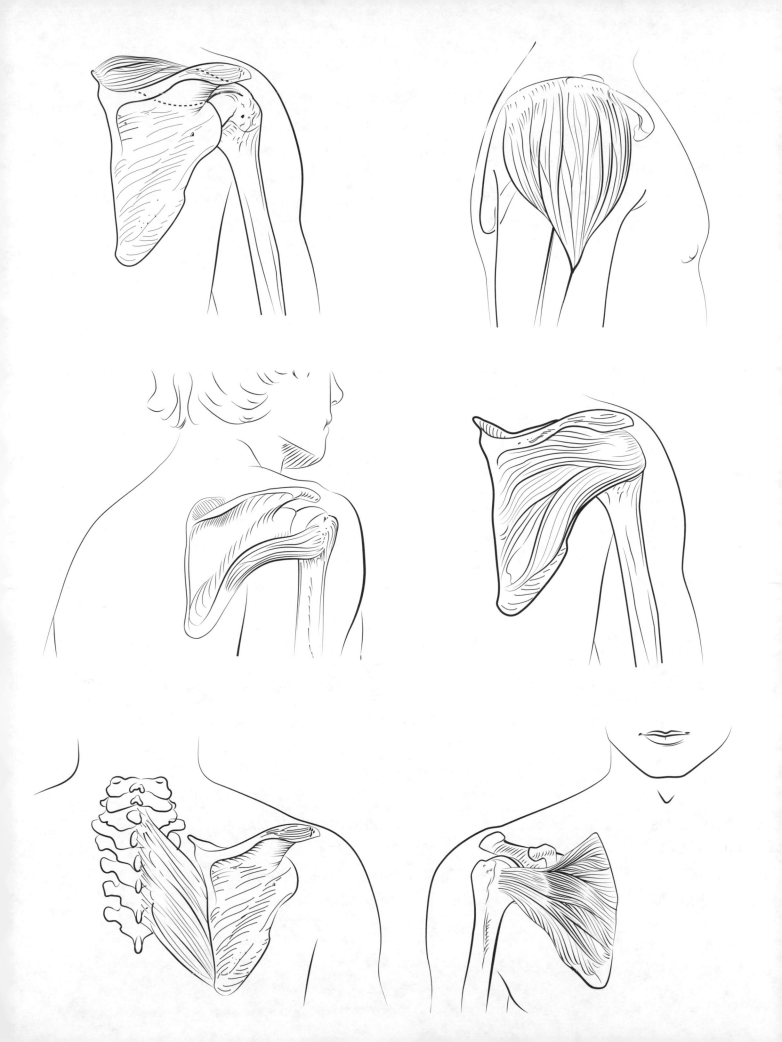

DELTOID

O: Clavicle, acromion, and spine of scapula

I: Deltoid tuberosity

A: Abducts, flexes, extends medially, and laterally rotates arm

SUPRASPINATUS

O: Supraspinous fossa

I: Greater tubercle of humerus

A: Abducts arm, stabilizes shoulder

INFRASPINATUS

O: Infraspinous fossa

I: Greater tubercle of humerus

A: Extends, laterally rotates arm, stabilizes shoulder

TERES MINOR

O: Axillary border of scapula

I: Greater tubercle of humerus

A: Extends, laterally rotates, adducts arm, stabilizes shoulder

SUBSCAPULARIS

O: Subscapular fossa

I: Lesser tubercle of humerus

A: Extends, medially rotates arm, stabilizes shoulder

RHOMBOIDEUS MAJOR

O: T1–T4

I: Inferior, medial border of scapula

A: Adducts scapula

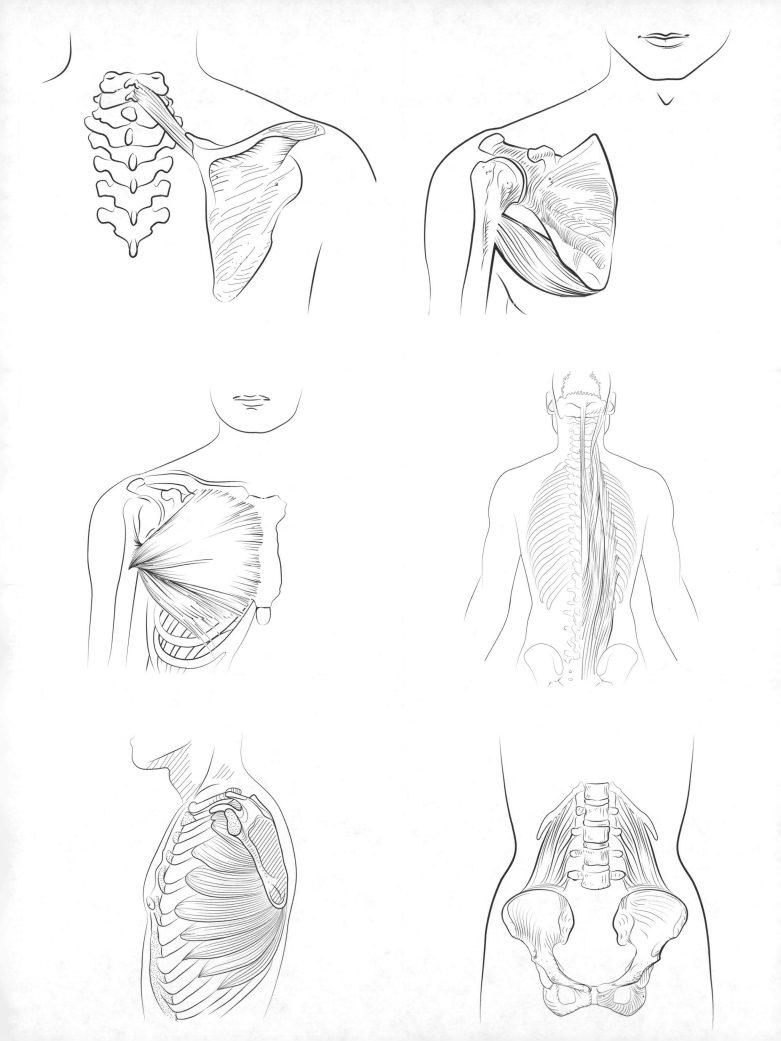

TERES MAJOR

O: Axillary border of scapula

I: Crest of lesser tubercle of humerus

A: Extends, adducts, medially rotates arm

RHOMBOIDEUS MINOR

O: Ligamentum nuchae, C6–C7

I: Superior, medial border of scapula

A: Adducts scapula

ERECTOR SPINAE: (SPINALIS, LONGISSIMUS, ILIOCOSTALIS) AND MULTIFIDUS

O: Vertebral column, ilium, sacrum, ribs

I: Ribs, vertebral column, occipital bone, temporal bone

A: Rotates and extends vertebral column and head

PECTORALIS MAJOR

O: Clavicle, sternum, and ribs 1–7

I: Crest of greater tubercle of humerus

A: Adducts, flexes, and rotates arm medially

QUADRATUS LUMBORUM

O: Iliac crest, lower lumbar vertebrae

I: T12, L1–L4, rib 12

A: Abducts vertebral column, depresses rib 12

SERRATUS ANTERIOR

O: Ribs 1–8 or 9

I: Vertebral border of scapula

A: Abducts scapula

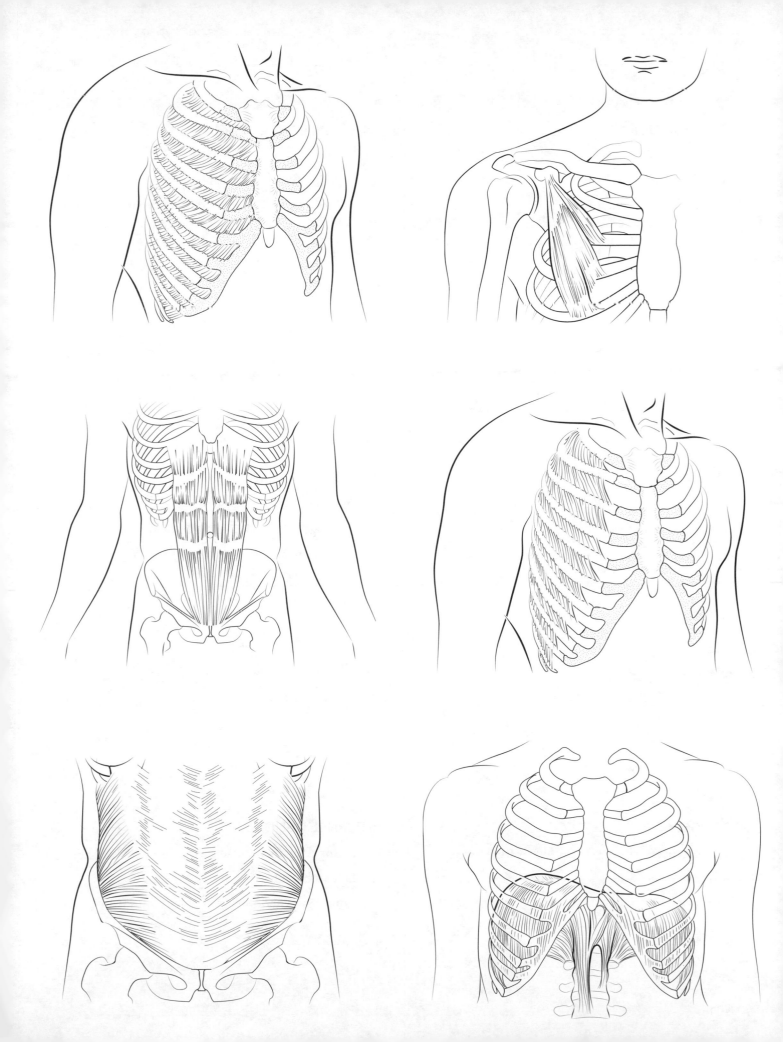

PECTORALIS MINOR

O: Ribs 3–5

I: Coracoid process of scapula

A: Depresses scapula, elevates ribs 3–5

INTERNAL INTERCOSTALIS

O: Inferior margin of ribs 1–11

I: Superior margin of ribs 2–12

A: Depresses ribs (decreases thoracic volume)

EXTERNAL INTERCOSTALIS

O: Inferior margin of ribs 1–11

I: Superior margin of ribs 2–12

A: Elevates ribs (increases thoracic volume)

RECTUS ABDOMINIS

O: Symphysis pubis and pubic crest

I: Cartilages of ribs 5–7 and xiphoid process

A: Flexes lumbar vertebrae, compresses abdomen

DIAPHRAGM

O: Xiphoid process, ribs 10–12, lumbar vertebrae

I: Central tendon

A: Inspiration

INTERNAL OBLIQUE

O: Inguinal ligament, iliac crest

I: Linea alba, inferior 4 ribs

A: Compresses abdomen, laterally rotates trunk

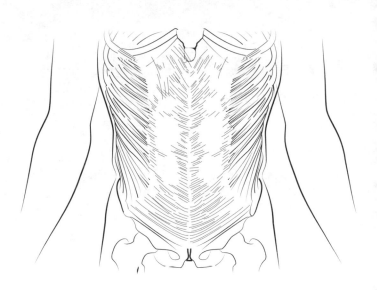
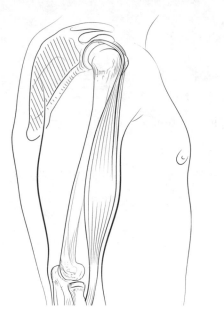
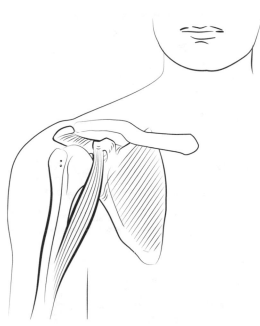
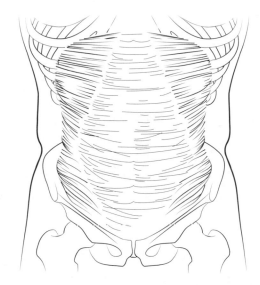
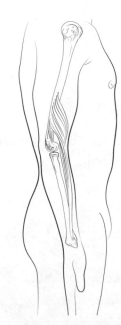
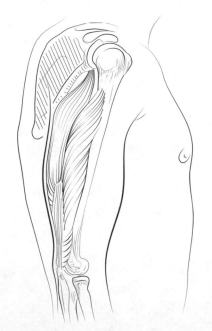

EXTERNAL OBLIQUE

O: Ribs 5–12

I: Iliac crest, inguinal ligament, linea alba

A: Compresses abdomen, laterally rotates trunk

BICEPS BRACHII

O: Supraglenoid tubercle, coracoid process

I: Radial tuberosity

A: Flexes arm, flexes and laterally rotates forearm (supinates hand)

TRANSVERSUS ABDOMINIS

O: Iliac crest, inguinal ligament, ribs 7–12

I: Linea alba, pubis

A: Compresses abdomen, laterally rotates trunk

CORACOBRACHIALIS

O: Coracoid process

I: Medial shaft of humerus

A: Adducts and flexes arm

TRICEPS BRACHII

O: Infraglenoid tuberosity of scapula, posterior surface of humerus

I: Olecranon process

A: Adducts arm, extends arm and forearm

BRACHIORADIALIS

O: Lateral supracondylar ridge of humerus

I: Styloid process of radius

A: Flexes forearm

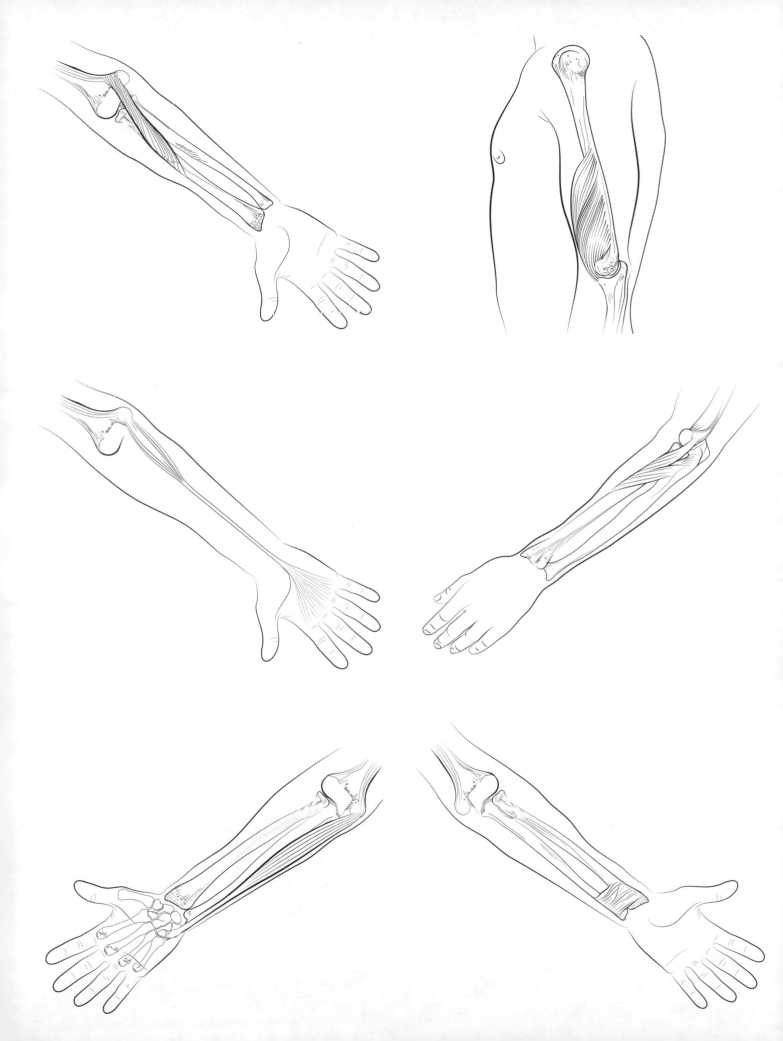

BRACHIALIS

O: Anterior, distal humerus

I: Coronoid process of ulna

A: Flexes forearm

PRONATOR TERES

O: Medial epicondyle of humerus, coronoid process of ulna

I: Lateral radius

A: Flexes and medially rotates forearm (pronates hand)

SUPINATOR

O: Lateral epicondyle of humerus, proximal ulna

I: Proximal shaft of radius

A: Supinates hand

PALMARIS LONGUS

O: Medial epicondyle of humerus

I: Palmar aponeurosis

A: Flexes hand

PRONATOR QUADRATUS

O: Anterior, distal ulna

I: Anterior, distal radius

A: Medially rotates forearm (pronates hand)

FLEXOR CARPI ULNARIS

O: Medial epicondyle of humerus olecranon and proximal ulna

I: Pisiform, hamate, metacarpal 5

A: Flexes and adducts hand

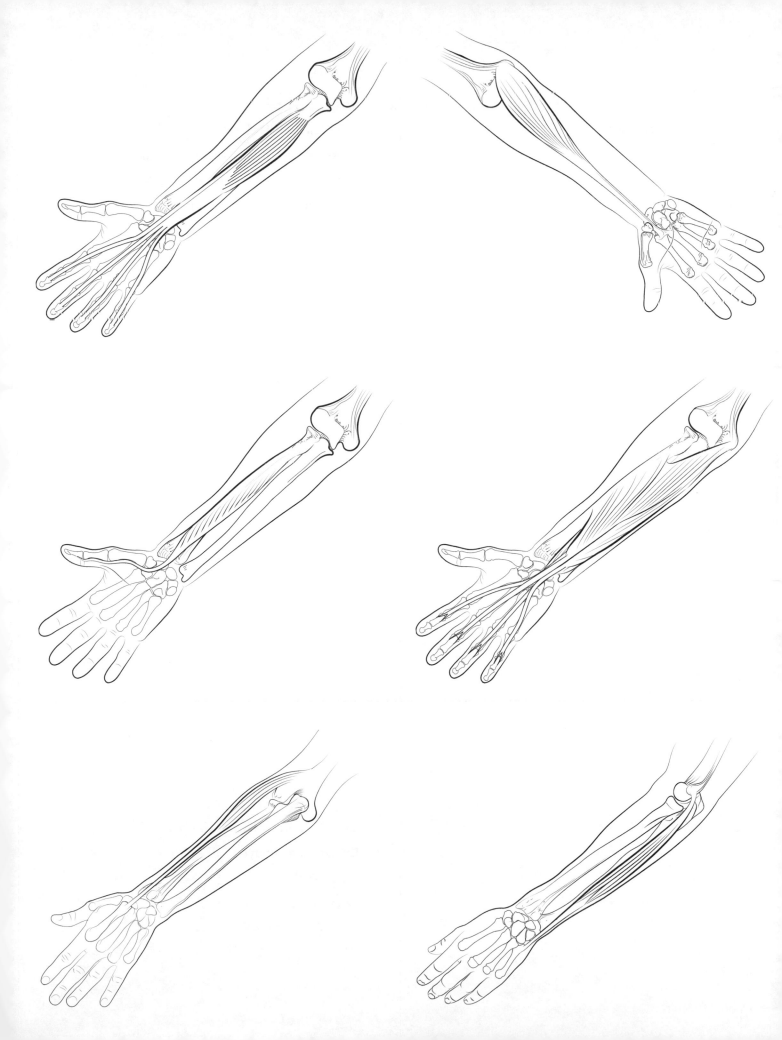

FLEXOR CARPI RADIALIS

O: Medial epicondyle of humerus

I: Metacarpals 2 and 3

A: Flexes and abducts hand

FLEXOR DIGITORUM PROFUNDUS

O: Proximal ulna, interosseus membrane

I: Anterior distal phalanges of digits 2–5

A: Flexes phalanges 2–5, flexes hand

FLEXOR DIGITORUM SUPERFICIALIS

O: Medial epicondyle of humerus, coronoid process of ulna, proximal shaft of radius

I: Middle phalanges of digits 2–5

A: Flexes proximal and middle phalanges of digits 2–5, flexes hand

FLEXOR POLLICIS LONGUS

O: Anterior aspect of radius and interosseus membrane

I: Distal phalanx of thumb (pollex)

A: Flexes thumb

EXTENSOR CARPI ULNARIS

O: Lateral epicondyle of humerus, posterior ulna

I: Metacarpal 5

A: Extends and adducts hand

EXTENSOR CARPI RADIALIS LONGUS

O: Lateral supracondylar ridge of humerus

I: Metacarpal 2

A: Extends and abducts hand

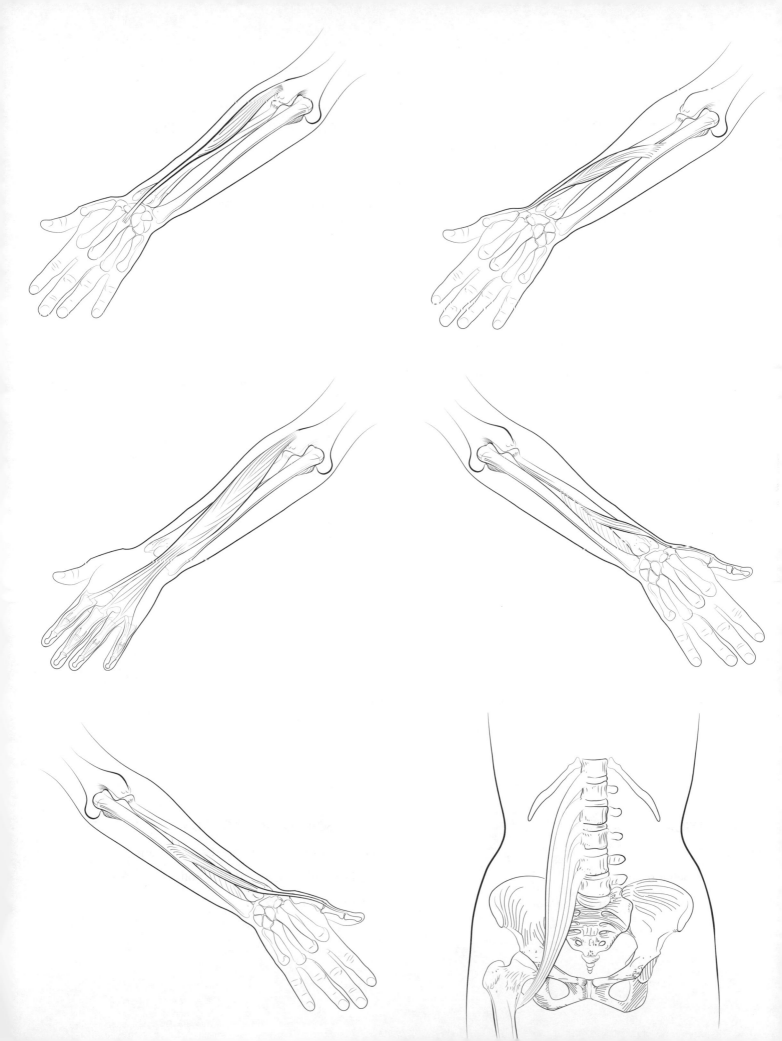

ABDUCTOR POLLICIS LONGUS

O: Posterior radial and ulnar surface, interosseus membrane

I: Metacarpal 1

A: Abducts and extends thumb

EXTENSOR CARPI RADIALIS BREVIS

O: Lateral epicondyle of humerus

I: Metacarpal 3

A: Extends and abducts hand

EXTENSOR POLLICIS BREVIS

O: Posterior radius, interosseus membrane

I: Proximal phalanx of thumb (pollex)

A: Extends thumb

EXTENSOR DIGITORUM

O: Lateral epicondyle of humerus

I: Middle and distal phalanges of digits 2–5

A: Extends all phalanges of digits 2–5, extends hand

PSOAS MAJOR

O: T12, L1–5

I: Lesser trochanter of femur

A: Flexes thigh and lumbar vertebrae

EXTENSOR POLLICIS LONGUS

O: Posterior ulna, interosseus membrane

I: Distal phalanx of thumb (pollex)

A: Extends thumb

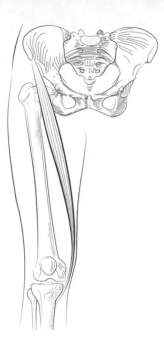

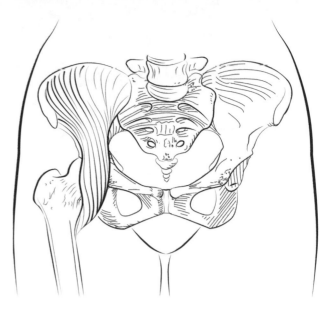

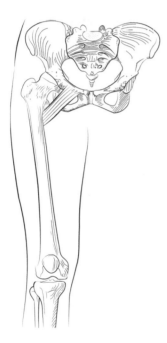

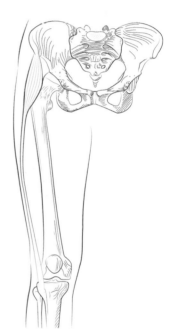

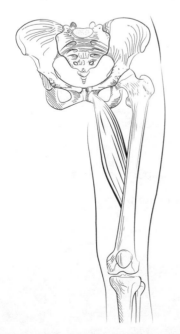

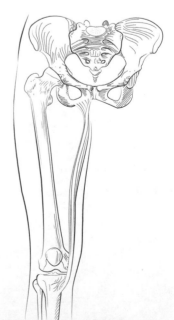

ILIACUS

O: Iliac fossa, sacrum

I: Lesser trochanter of femur

A: Flex thigh

SARTORIUS

O: Anterior superior iliac spine

I: Medial side of tibial tuberosity

A: Flexes and laterally rotates thigh, flexes leg

TENSOR FASCIAE LATAE

O: Anterior superior iliac spine

I: Lateral condyle of tibia by the iliotibial band

A: Flexes, medially rotates, and abducts thigh

PECTINEUS

O: Pubis

I: Proximal, posterior femur

A: Adducts and laterally rotates thigh

GRACILIS

O: Pubis

I: Proximal portion of medial tibia

A: Adducts thigh, flexes leg

ADDUCTOR LONGUS

O: Pubis

I: Middle linea aspera of femur

A: Adducts and laterally rotates thigh

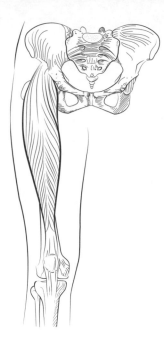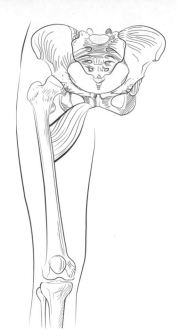

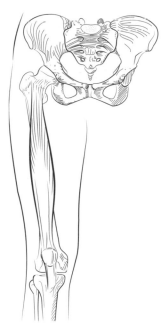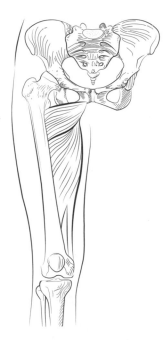

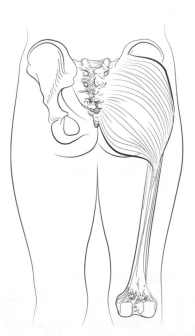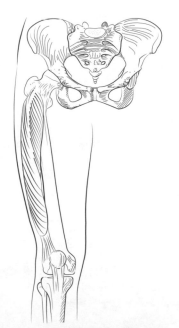

ADDUCTOR BREVIS

O: Pubis

I: Proximal linea aspera of femur

A: Adducts and laterally rotates thigh

RECTUS FEMORIS

O: Anterior inferior iliac spine

I: Tibial tuberosity

A: Flexes thigh, extends leg

ADDUCTOR MAGNUS

O: Ischium and pubis

I: Linea aspera and adductor tubercle of femur

A: Adducts, flexes, extends, and laterally rotates thigh

VASTUS INTERMEDIUS

O: Anterior and lateral part of femur

I: Tibial tuberosity

A: Extends leg

VASTUS LATERALIS

O: Greater trochanter and linea aspera of femur

I: Tibial tuberosity

A: Extends leg

GLUTEUS MAXIMUS

O: Lateral surface of ilium, sacrum, coccyx

I: Lateral condyle of tibia by lateral fascia, gluteal tuberosity of femur

A: Extends, abducts, and laterally rotates thigh

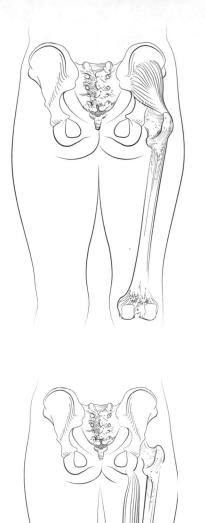
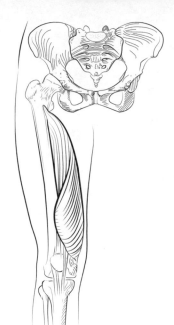
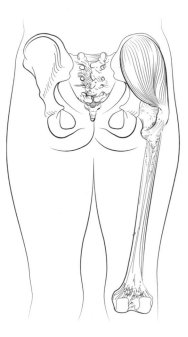
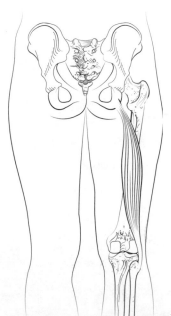
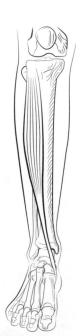

VASTUS MEDIALIS

O: Linea aspera of femur

I: Tibial tuberosity

A: Extends leg

GLUTEUS MINIMUS

O: Outer ilium

I: Greater trochanter of femur

A: Medially rotates and abducts thigh

GLUTEUS MEDIUS

O: Outer ilium

I: Greater trochanter of femur

A: Medially rotates and abducts thigh

SEMITENDINOSUS

O: Ischial tuberosity

I: Medial tibia near tibial tuberosity

A: Extends thigh, flexes and medially rotates leg

BICEPS FEMORIS

O: Ischial tuberosity, distal linea aspera of femur

I: Head of fibula, lateral tibia

A: Extends thigh, flexes and laterally rotates leg

TIBIALIS ANTERIOR

O: Lateral tibia

I: First metatarsal and medial cuneiform

A: Dorsiflexes and inverts foot

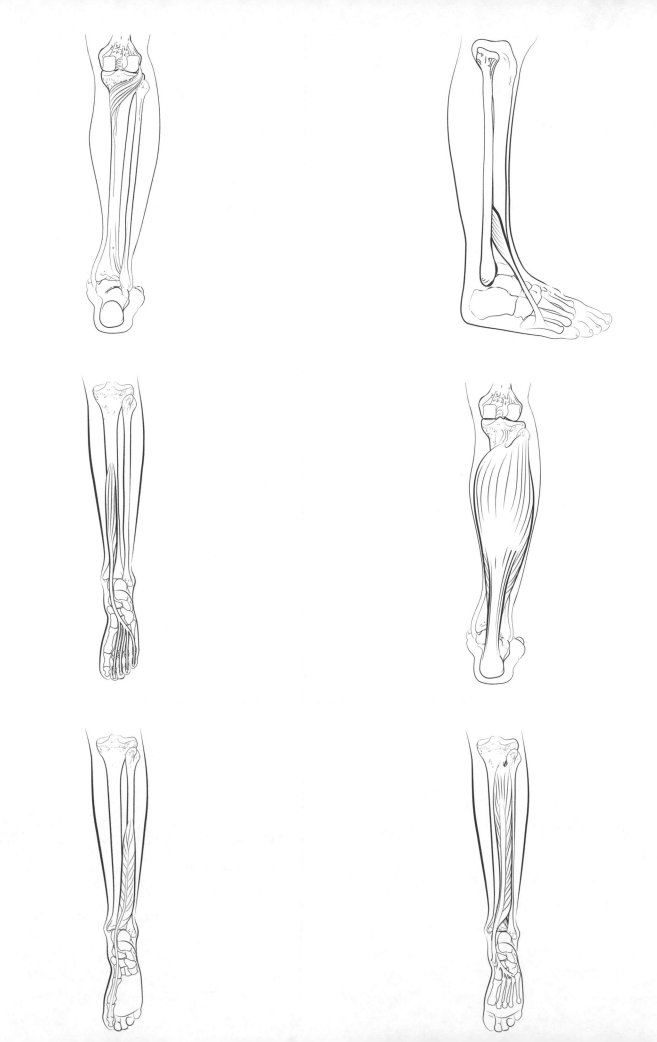

FIBULARIS TERTIUS

O: Distal fibula, interosseous membrane

I: Superior aspect of metatarsal 5

A: Dorsiflexes and everts foot

POPLITEUS

O: Lateral condyle of femur

I: Proximal tibia

A: Flexes and medially rotates leg

SOLEUS

O: Posterior tibia and fibula

I: Calcaneus

A: Plantar flexes foot

FLEXOR DIGITORUM LONGUS

O: Posterior tibia

I: Distal phalanges of digits 2–5

A: Flexes toes, plantar flexes and inverts foot

TIBIALIS POSTERIOR

O: Posterior tibia and fibula

I: Metatarsals 2–4, navicular, cuneiforms and cuboid

A: Plantar flexes and inverts foot

FLEXOR HALLUCIS LONGUS

O: Middle fibula

I: Distal phalanx of hallux

A: Flexes hallux, plantar flexes and inverts foot

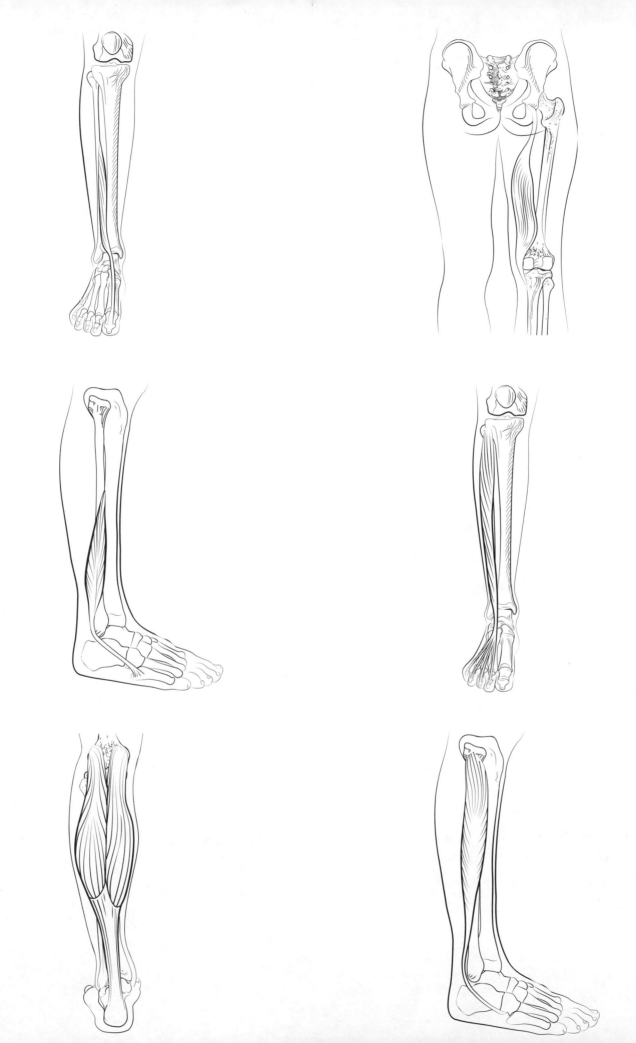

SEMIMEMBRANOSUS

O: Ischial tuberosity

I: Medial tibial condyle

A: Extends thigh, flexes and medially rotates leg

EXTENSOR HALLUCIS LONGUS

O: Medial shaft of fibula, interosseous membrane

I: Distal phalanx of hallux (first digit)

A: Extends hallux, dorsiflexes foot and inverts foot

EXTENSOR DIGITORUM LONGUS

O: Lateral tibial condyle, shaft of fibula

I: Middle and distal phalanges of digits 2–5

A: Extends digits 2–5, dorsiflexes and everts foot

FIBULARIS BREVIS

O: Fibula

I: Metatarsal 5

A: Plantar flexes and everts foot

FIBULARIS LONGUS

O: Proximal fibula, lateral condyle of tibia

I: First metatarsal, medial cuneiform

A: Plantar flexes and everts foot

GASTROCNEMIUS

O: Lateral and medial condyles of femur

I: Calcaneus

A: Flexes leg, plantar flexes foot